"This even works for a food addict. You can do it, I did"

FAT NO MORE!
THE BOOK OF HOPE FOR LOSING WEIGHT

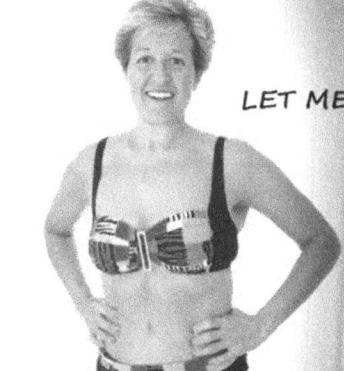

LET ME HELP YOU!

- THE BOOK OF HOPE
- ENJOY BEING THIN
- DON'T WAIT, START THE "CURE"
- NO MORE FAILED DIETS

ONE EX-OBESE WOMAN'S STRUGGLES AND SUCCESS

DR. SUSAN R. CUSHING

╫RICHER Press
An Imprint of Richer Life, LLC

RICHER Press is a full service, specialty Trade publisher whose sole goal is to *shape thoughts and change lives for the better*. All of the books, eBooks and digital media we publish, distribute and market embrace our commitment to help maximize opportunities for personal growth and professional achievement.

To learn more visit
www.richerlifellc.com.

Publisher's Disclaimer

This book does not provide medical advice.

Causes for being overweight or obese vary from person to person. Whether genetic or environmental, it should be noted that food intake, rates of metabolism and levels of exercise and physical exertion vary from person to person. This means weight loss results will also vary from person to person. No individual result should be seen as typical.

The information, including but not limited to, text, graphics, images and other material, contained in this book is for educational and inspirational purposes only. The content is not intended in any way as a substitute for professional medical advice, diagnosis or treatment. Always seek the advice of your physician or other qualified health care provider with any questions you may have regarding a medical condition or treatment and before undertaking a new health care regimen, and never disregard professional medical advice or delay in seeking it because of something you have read in this book.

Copyright © 2014 by Susan R. Cushing

Published by ✠RICHER Press
An Imprint of Richer Life, LLC

4600 E. Washington Street, Suite 300, Phoenix, Arizona 85034
www.richerlifellc.com

Cover Design: RICHER Media USA

No part of this publication may be reproduced, stored in a retrieval system, or transmitted in any form or by any means, electronic, mechanical, photocopying, recording, scanning, or otherwise, except as permitted under Section 107 or 108 of the 1976 United States Copyright Act, without prior written permission of the publisher.

Library of Congress Cataloging-in-Publications Data

Fat No More!
The Book of Hope For Losing Weight
Susan R. Cushing
p.   cm.

1. Self Help   2. Weight Loss   3. Inspiration
ISBN 978-0-9899001-7-1
(pbk : alk. Paper)

2014935145

ISBN 13: 978-0-9899001-7-1
ISBN 10: 0-9899001-7-1

Text set is Adobe Garamond

PRINTED IN THE UNITED STATES OF AMERICA

March 2014

CONTENTS

Acknowledgements — 11

Personal Note to My Readers — 13

Introduction — 15
Is it a Coincidence or a Power in the Universe?

Chapter 1 — Childhood History of Obesity — 19

Chapter 2 — Consequences of Childhood Obesity — 29

Chapter 3 — To the Struggling Food Addict — 41

Chapter 4 — My Personal Experience with Joining FA: Food Addicts in Recovery — 45

Chapter 5 — My Reflections on Obesity and Finding HCG — 57

Chapter 6 — In Summary: What I Have Learned — 63

Chapter 7 — A Glimmer of Hope for Me — 67

Chapter 8 — Deciding to Try "The Weight Loss Cure" Program — 69

Chapter 9	The Weight Loss Cure	75
Chapter 10	Cleanse Day: Diet Steak Day	103
Chapter 11	Colonics	105
Chapter 12	Constipation	109
Chapter 13	Thoughts on Exercise and the Rebounder	113
Chapter 14	Testing My Limits, My Metabolism and My Hypothalamus	115
Chapter 15	Just Say No! Combining My FA Structure with "The Weight Loss Cure" Program	123
Chapter 16	Enjoying Success with a Reset Hypothalamus	129
Chapter 17	Thoughts on Mood and Depression	133
Chapter 18	After Weight Loss	137
Chapter 19	Cosmetic Surgery: The Why, How and the Process	143
Chapter 20	Choosing a Cosmetic Surgeon	151
Chapter 21	Key Journal Notes Regarding My Surgical Experience	161

Chapter 22	Dealing with Insomnia: Complicated by Food Addiction	189
Chapter 23	Regrets	193
Summary		197

About the Author	199
Author's Disclaimer	201
Bibliography, Resources and References	203
Overview of Susan's Lifelong Weight Challenge	205

Acknowledgements

I have many thanks to say and many people that have empowered me and given me encouragement in my process, which has allowed me to write this book.

- ❖ I would like to acknowledge Kevin Trudeau for his excellent, controversial book, "The Weight Loss Cure." Kevin wrote his book and offered hope to thousands, including me. It was his book which was the final missing piece that gave me the solution to getting rid of my excess weight. I also appreciate his many wonderful suggestions and additions to my health regimen.

- ❖ Special acknowledgements go to A.T.W. Simeons for his manuscript, "Pounds and Inches: A New Approach to Obesity," where he shares his discoveries and treatment for weight loss.

- ❖ My sincerest gratitude and deep love goes to my best friend and supporter in my life and in all my endeavors, my companion and loving husband of 29 years, Curt.

- ❖ To the FA 12 Step Program of recovery, the founders of AA (on which FA is modeled), and the co-founders of FA.

- ❖ To HCG Medical and all their wonderful staff.

- ❖ To my supportive friend, Alice, who was always there for me during good times and challenging times, and has helped me grow as a woman.

- ❖ To my FA sponsor, Rachel, who has always given me unconditional love and spiritual guidance.

- ❖ To my colonic therapist, Pam.
- ❖ To the Amber Waves Health Food Store.
- ❖ To my massage therapist, Carolynne.
- ❖ To my cosmetic surgeon, Dr. Fater.
- ❖ I also want to thank my fabulous support system including Camille, Janice, Hawley, Chris, Joy, and Kim. Also to my many sponsors in my recovery programs, and many others that were there for me…helping me day by day. This was a period in my life that was difficult and seemed more than I could handle alone.
- ❖ To myself for my persistence and never giving up and believing that there was a solution.
- ❖ To all the resources that helped this once 205 pound woman reach her goals.

A Personal Note To My Readers

When I read Kevin Trudeau's book, I tried using all the suggested websites including his, but became very frustrated. I was unable to locate or reach any of the specific referrals listed in his book. It seemed to me that for some reason, Kevin had hidden it well and I would have to pay to join his website to get the needed information. After many days of research and what felt like wasted effort, I was finally was able to locate a very helpful company. They were extremely knowledgeable and encouraging. I chose to turn my health issues and desires over to their care in order find the best medical answers and to achieve my goals.

To save you, my desperate readers, any more time and grief, I am offering this information to you, i.e. HCG Medical.

I have since learned that there are other companies and alternative medical practitioners that will guide you and help you with the HCG process for weight loss.

I do not know if what Kevin states at the bottom of page 104 of his book is true: that "the drug companies, the food companies, the government and the media do not want you to know the truth about this "obesity cure breakthrough." However, I do know that when I visited any medical person I knew, including many MD's and specialists, none of them offered any successful solution to help my weight problem. None of them offered anything of use, concerning my specific metabolism issue and many did not believe in this HCG regimen nor would they even suggest that it could help. The concern that many of them had was that it could hurt me.

I have spent many years of my own personal research trying out all kinds of trial and error suggestions and nothing has worked as well for my problem as following this HCG process exactly as the book advised. It has been absolutely amazing. You must try this if you have tried everything else and cannot get your weight to a "healthy, normal" level. Before totally giving up and accepting that you will ALWAYS be fat, commit yourself to try the "Weight Loss Cure."

Introduction

Is it a Coincidence or a Power in the Universe?

Over the years I have attended numerous workshops and studied extensively on the concepts of "Universal Abundance", God, Higher Power, Spirit and Universal Energy. I have been told and have come to believe the following statement: "the Universe provides". Depending on your own personal religious and spiritual beliefs, you could replace the word "Universe" with "God," "Higher Power," "The Great Spirit," "Spirit", "Universal Energy" or even "The Force".

From my experience, I have seen that when I am fully committed to do the legwork and am ready and willing to proceed, "The Universe" seems to allow things to come together to give me what I need and really want. It seems that I am ultimately led to what I ask for and what is good for me.

This phenomenon of abundance happened to me while searching for an answer to get thin. After I had tried everything I could think of and was at my wit's end and fully ready to do "whatever it would take" to get the fat off of my body and be thin, two friends suggested that I read the book titled, "The Secret." In one of the chapters of this book the author, Jack Canfield, said that if we could imagine and believe that we could have anything we wanted, and wanted it badly enough, we could get it.

Soon after reading that statement, three of my dearest friends suggested that I read Kevin Trudeau's book, "The Weight Loss Cure". Since a total of three people had mentioned his book within a very short period of time, I felt directed to get the book and read it. Surprisingly enough, this book opened up the door for my personal and final solution for my weight loss dilemma. Ultimately, it allowed my entire world to become alive again. I lost my excess weight and all the "stubborn fat." I felt that I had experienced my own personal miracle. I would say that when I was ready and open minded enough, "The Universe" ultimately led me to what I desired most. I am sure glad that I was listening and willing to follow.

Are you ready and willing to believe and follow?

As you read through this book you will find references to a "Higher Power" and the Twelve Steps of recovery.

I am a recovering member of Food Addicts in Recovery, referred to a FA. This is a spiritual program for food addiction based on the principles of Alcoholics Anonymous. By working through the Twelve Steps outlined in this program, I have been able to find a Power greater than myself that I can utilize to keep my food addiction neutralized one day at a time. I believe that this "Power' or "Universal Energy" or "Spirit" has led me to Kevin Trudeau's book, "The Weight Loss Cure", just when I was desperate enough. At that time, I was ready to give up and surrender all I thought I knew and be willing to try something totally different. I do not know if any of my readers believe in or need an unending source of strength, but for me it has made a huge difference. This "undefined Power" has allowed me to turn my view of the world around, thereby making my entire life function more smoothly and serenely.

I have no answer as to how this "energy force" works for me or for anyone else. I just know that all my experiences keep proving to me that I need it and have to use it daily. I have learned over and over, the hard way, that whenever I try and be totally self-reliant and "go it alone', I invariable end up getting frustrated and spinning my wheels and looking once again for help from others and from outside resources. As a recovering food addict, I can sometimes feel like a "relief seeking missile", where I am out searching for something to appease my desires and placate my inner angst. For me this 'Power greater than myself' has helped me turn that around, calm down and even feel fulfilled in unexpected ways.

If you already use this "Power", I'm sure you understand what I am saying. However, if you have never considered this, I suggest you try it and see for yourself if it doesn't somehow lighten your load and make your life a little easier.

When I was young, my peers mocked me because my weight made me look disfigured and I could not wear any of the clothes other children wore. Basically, I looked fat and frumpy.

CHAPTER 1

My History of Obesity

I have always felt like my body did not function like most other people's bodies. My metabolism seemed sluggish and I had lower energy levels compared to my peers. I seemed drawn to flour and sugar, yet when I ate it, I always felt hungrier and had to eat more of it. After I ate these foods I would immediately feel bloated and a bit groggy, but then I would feel pacified and somewhat euphoric. I noticed that even when I would eat less than my peers, I would get fat. When I would overeat, I seemed to gain more weight than the amount of calories consumed. Then when I was put on a diet, I always lost less weight than my peers on the same diet and I could never seem to lose all my excess weight, no matter what I did. I would try over and over, to no avail. My doctor's actually told me that I "must be cheating", but I knew when I was being honest and when I was not. I felt betrayed by those who were supposed to be helping me and eventually I would give up. This, I repeated over and over again.

When I was young, my peers mocked me because my weight made me look disfigured and I could not wear any of the clothes other children wore. Basically, I looked fat and frumpy. My mother tried to help and took me to a doctor, but he did not believe me when I honestly told him what I was eating. When the doctor intimated that I was lying about my food, I felt betrayed and hopeless. I really wanted to lose the excess weight and be thin like my peers, but his judgment left me feeling alone and powerless to do anything about it.

For most of my life, I felt like I was in a paradox, my own "Catch 22". I would go on a diet and no matter how hard I tried, I was unable to reach a realistic goal and get all my excess weight off. The paradox was that as much as I wanted to be thin, I was also compelled to eat to feel better. My childish response to this failure would be to give up by hiding out from people and turning to food: first as my comfort and later as my "lover". However, I also thought of food as my constant enemy, because I fought it all the time and yet gave in when I would feel defeated.

In 1977, when I was 20 years old, I found my first real hope with OA, Overeaters Anonymous, a 12 Step program for Compulsive Overeaters, where I learned that I had a definite adverse reaction to all sugar and flour products. I followed their food plan and did what I was told to do by my sponsor and mentors, but I still felt different. I seemed to struggle most days not to eat anything extra and I felt obsessed and afraid of food most of the time. No matter how hard I tried, I remained heavier than the rest of my fellow OA members. I did have success with some weight loss, but I could never get off the last 25 pounds of excess weight. I was 5 foot 2 and ½ inches tall and my weight loss stopped when I reached between 140-145 pounds, even eating 1000 calories per day.

It seemed to me, that others in OA were out living their lives, while I spent most of my time and energy just trying to get thin and never achieving it. When I couldn't reach a reasonable goal weight but everyone else around me could, it affected my already low self-esteem and added to my poor body image.

In 1996, around age 41, I found the diet regimen using the medications Fen-Phen, (Fenfluramine-Phentermine), where I had really good physical results and began to feel better than I ever had before. I was happy, had lots of energy, reached 112 pounds and felt like a sexy woman ready to conquer the world. When I reached my goal and therefore stopped taking the pills, my food compulsion and desire to eat returned. I was hungry a lot of the time and I eventually returned to eating excessively. My cravings for and my addiction to sugar and flour returned, I regained the lost weight and I reached the lowest emotional point I had ever felt until then. I was feeling pretty defeated and almost ready to give up on my life and just wait to die! I had heard the expression: "It's always the darkest before the dawn". And so it was for me!

After sinking to that very low point in 1998, I unexpectedly found FA, Food Addict's in Recovery Anonymous, and a glimmer of hope surfaced. Since I felt extremely desperate with nothing to lose, I gave up what I thought I knew and followed exactly what was suggested. I was committed to do whatever I had to, wanting to believe that I could have the same results everyone else in FA had experienced.

I entered the FA program at 175 pounds and eventually reached 125 pounds. It took me two full years to reach this goal: much more time than anyone else I knew in the program. Soon after reaching this goal weight, I began having trouble keeping my weight stable and it went up and down. At this time, I also lost my menstrual period and my Gynecologist prescribed Birth Control pills that had a small amount of Estrogen added. Within two weeks, I had regained 12 pounds and became very upset. My doctor was shocked and told me to stop taking the pills and said as soon as I stopped taking the pills, I would lose the extra pounds. However, after one month, my weight was still creeping up.

Being a relatively young woman and not having a menstrual period, I was concerned about my medical health. I wanted medical help to get my menstrual period back and to lose the regained weight. Since I had lost confidence in my Gynecologist, I decided to try a Naturopath. The Naturopath was able to help me get back my menstrual period, but she could not help me get my extra weight off. She told me that I had a metabolism issue, not just a weight problem, and it was most likely due to something abnormal or unbalanced in my Pituitary or my Hypothalamus. She said she had a few patients like me and unfortunately medical science did not have any tests, yet, to determine where our problems originated from or how to treat them.

As you might expect, I was extremely frustrated and upset and determined to get some medical help that I felt had to be "out there", somewhere. All in all, I went to 3 primary care doctors, 4 Endocrinologists, 2 Nutritionists, a Naturopath, 2 Chiropractors, an Acupuncturist, and many types of therapists; traditional and alternative. I followed all their suggestions and even took their suggested remedies and antidepressants for relief. I tried many "safe" over the counter diet drugs, "Internet cures", tried hair analysis", herbal supplements like "St John's Wort, and all types of vitamins. I tried everything I could think of or what proclaimed to offer any help, but nothing worked or even made any sense. As you might imagine, my desperation increased.

This was the state I was in while I was searching for anything to help me and found: "The Weight Loss Cure". When I read this book by Kevin Trudeau, the unsolved puzzle came together. I identified with everything completely and it all felt true for me. I began to feel a spark of hope which I had not felt once my weight started coming on again from October 2002 to Jan 2006. That was when my weight had jumped from 125 pounds to 150 pounds while I was following an 800-1000 calorie food plan and my continued daily exercise on the treadmill.

As I remember it now, I think what made me so angry was how all the doctors and practitioners, kept telling me: "Accept yourself", because none of them could actually help me. They just did not understand. It appeared to me that since they had no answers, they felt frustrated themselves, and just gave up on me. I also found it interesting that many of them seemed to have also given up on their own obesity problem and were just offering me their personal answer of resignation.

I remember thinking: "How easy for them to say "Accept yourself", when either they had never had any trouble with their weight, or they just don't care about their overweight status and have given up trying to lose any". Although I felt depressed, wanted to give up, had lost hope, felt like I looked like a "swollen balloon", and was afraid to eat anything for fear of gaining more weight, somehow I never gave up completely! I called myself a survivor and I just kept searching.

I wonder just how many other survivors are out there who are just like me, looking for an answer to their prayers. How many of you have tried just about everything, each time with hope of success, only to not lose weight and fail again? I'll bet there are many.

For me, as soon as I read Kevin's book and Dr. Simeone's manuscript, which is alluded to as the basis of his book, I knew I had found my answer. A real cure was actually promised!

I am sure many of you can relate to what I had been doing and have even felt the same. I am speaking about spending most of my life desperately trying to look and feel normal within my own body. From young adulthood on, I had felt like a caricature of what a woman should look like. I had a body that was shaped so very different from most girls my age. I felt like a "stuffed sausage"; my upper arms looked swollen, my knees were fatty, and my thighs, hips and derriere were fat. My inner thighs sagged and would rub together when I walked, which caused painful sores and wore away my pants. It limited any and all exercise or recreational activity that I tried. I had to walk and carry myself around differently because of all my fat. No amount of dieting ever changed the sagging, the "cellulite", or the excess fat on my body.

When I followed the FA program as diligently and honestly as was possible, I reached a point where my addiction was gone and food became only fuel to live. I no longer ate for pure emotional reasons. This was a huge accomplishment for me and I felt that now all I had to do was maintain my weight like others in FA were doing.

However as I alluded to above, my weight began to creep back on, just as I had experienced many times before, no matter what food plan I had been following. When it happened to me in FA, I began to gain an average of 1 pound a month, until I had gained 30 pounds and saw no end in sight. I was terrified and scared beyond belief. I was horrified that it could be happening to me again. All my childhood and adult feelings of shame and humiliation came back with a vengeance. I began to question everything I was doing. I even asked myself: "Was I eating and forgetting? Was I sleep-eating like I had done in my past? I started to feel like I was losing my sanity.

Fortunately, I believed in myself and how I was living and I had enough "Recovery" in FA that I knew I had NOT cheated, and had been totally honest and clean with my food. I had no doubt that I was Abstinent and Sober as we say in the 12 Step program. It also helped that my husband acted like a reality test for me. He had been watching me closely and was a witness to my horrifying truth and reaffirmed to me that I was living honestly and not "cheating".

I went to any and all FA members who had had any difficulty losing weight, but had succeeded, the "FA winners" as they are lovingly referred to. I asked for their help and took any new suggestions, trying anything that had worked for them. To my dismay, it was all to no avail, for no matter how many different food plans I tried, my weight would not budge and still kept slowly creeping up.

Unfortunately, many of these "supportive" FA members began to stop calling me and over time, most fell away from my world. I am sure many of them felt frustrated, since they couldn't do anything for me and felt overwhelmed by how sad and miserable I felt all the time. Their rejection left me with almost no one to call to share my frustrations or to get any suggestions as to how to keep on going. I understood that many of them were probably confused and fearful of what was happening to me, and some even judged me and assumed I was eating and lying or just not being completely honest. The last reason felt the worst for me. It made me feel so angry, and caused me to become self-deprecating and feeling devastated. I turned inward once again and began to isolate myself.

Here was my one true "peer group", what I called my "family", the one place I had connected and felt like I had belonged, and yet they had judged me a liar. The hopelessness settled in full force. For me that was the ultimate betrayal. I was left alone again, "me against the world", to seek the answers to my truth. I had to find a way to trust in myself again and have hope.

I intuitively knew that there was something out of balance in my physical body and I just could not live with the consensus of opinion that I should just accept myself fat. One sponsor in FA even told me the spiritual answer was:" God doesn't want you fat, so for now just accept it and pray".

For me these were not helpful suggestions at the time. It proved to me the lack of true compassion and understanding of many of my FA peers. Since so many of them had been able to lose their excess weight so easily, they had no experience to draw on and they just "did not get it". I ended up feeling very angry towards them and pity for them. Yet, I could also identify with their frustration. What they did worked so well for them. So, why wasn't I having the same success?

It's very interesting how an image can stay with us for years and years and affect us in such a way as to cause us to make certain judgments. I remembered seeing a photo in a travel magazine, when I was just a teenager, of a very obese woman. I noticed that she had a very large derriere and she, too, had an odd distribution of fat. At the time my immature mind had judged her in a negative way while I also identified with her at the same time. I remember wondering if I would look like her for the rest of my life and felt terrible fear and distress. This added to my already poor body image and low self-esteem that I had connected so directly with my weight. Isn't it amazing how our minds work, and what affect certain pictures, memories or experiences have on us?

Being a very goal-driven woman, I have always had hopes and dreams for my life. That last affront of what seemed to me a betrayal by my peers, left me bereft of any hope, feeling useless, and totally powerless in my life. My internal reality was that I was just "surviving" as a fat woman, anyway, and not living a full, enjoyable life, so maybe I should finally just give up. I even began to question if I had ever really enjoyed my life.

That questioning got me to once again review my entire life's history. As I went through my life, I knew that one thing that always made life difficult for me was my constant nagging hunger, where I felt like I could never get "enough" food. However, I was always AFRAID of eating, because I did not want to get any fatter than I was. I felt constant shame mixed with guilt and fear that maybe everyone was right calling me a fat pig. I kept asking myself; "Why was I always so hungry and why was I was overweight and others were not, when I ate so much less that everyone I knew?" I understood intellectually that there were people with high metabolisms, but my BMI, (Basal Metabolic Index), tested by a nutritionist, said that I required 1250 calories a day just to keep my organs functioning, and I was eating only 1000 calories and gaining weight! It seemed so clear to me that something just did not measure up and something else had to be going on.

    Why could I never get my excess weight off? This seemed like "the million dollar question"! No one I ever heard of so far had any answers of merit, at least not until I read Dr. Simeone's transcript and Kevin Trudeau's book, "The Weight Loss Cure".

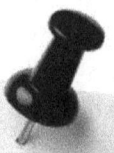

The way I viewed it, the weight and size of my body was not just a number on a scale to show the current status of my body, it was a judgment of my value as a person and a determination of whether I was acceptable to the world.

CHAPTER 2

Consequences of Childhood Obesity

Let me share some thoughts and experiences concerning obesity and my fat childhood, specifically. As everyone knows, although the world is changing, there are still many prejudices and stereotypes that remain in our society.

I have heard it said that obesity is truly the most longstanding and strongest held prejudice still held by a majority of people in our society today. All of my life's experiences agree with this. There are many who believe that thinness is a sign of beauty, strength, and power. I have spoken to many women that are thin and some that used to be fat and the consensus among them is that a certain power and prestige comes from being a thin woman in our culture. Fat people and fat women, specifically, are often judged as being ugly, stupid, even gluttons and considered to have no willpower.

While many of us can sympathize with people of other races, religions, social status and disabilities, many still seem to judge fat people harshly. They are looked down upon, called weak, and even berated for carrying excess weight. Statistically, fat people have less success getting good jobs, getting married in higher financially rewarding marriages and gaining acceptance into more prominent social circles. They even have less chance of getting into the most prestigious schools. Unfortunately they also have more medical problems that lead to more medical visits to an assortment of doctors. It's undeniable that for the most part, being fat is a detriment in many ways.

From the time I was a very young child in elementary school, I remember feeling entombed in a self-constructed prison of fat and isolation. I was resigned to it as being the way it was and always would be. As a result, I hated myself and felt the disdain from others.

The way I viewed it, the weight and size of my body was not just a number on a scale to show the current status of my body, it was a judgment of my value as a person and a determination of whether I was acceptable to the world. It determined whether others would consider me a glutton and fat and ugly, or attractive and worthy of their attention and kindness. My weight was a huge source of constant shame for me. The uncertainty I felt every day was whether I would be pitied, ignored or given a chance to be worthy of friendship and love.

Take a moment to imagine a society that looks down on all fat people, where the popular magazines and TV, mostly show beautiful, thin people as our role models and mentors. This visual media represent to the world the examples of how we should all be. Does this sound familiar to anyone? This was what I remember seeing when I was growing up.

Now put yourself in the mind and body of a small 8 and 1/2-year-old fat girl in the fourth grade. You are 50 pounds overweight and the fattest child in the class. Everyone can see your "disability" or "weight problem". Can you just imagine the immensity of this and what a child like that might be thinking, feeling, and believing about herself in a world focused on thinness. Can you even imagine her sense of shame and feelings of unworthiness?

This was exactly the learning I got and how I experienced what the world was like. When a young child at such an impressionable age has this type of input, it is carried through for the rest of their lives, coloring everything they think, do and believe. It determines how they learn to relate to the rest of the world.

Can you remember what it was like when you were in the 4th grade? Is there a memory that stands out for you more boldly than all the rest? Have you ever taken a moment and wondered what others seated next to you in class may have been thinking or feeling? Most of us never do, because we are all into our own little worlds and what we ourselves are experiencing at the moment. As parents well know, this is especially true of children and teenagers.

I have a photo from when I was in the 4th grade and went to a very orthodox school, the Lubavitz Yeshiva. My parents were not particularly religious, but my mother had heard that the school offered an excellent education and wanted her only daughter to have what she could only dream about. I realized when I got older; that it was a serious financial struggle and logistical challenge for my parents to send me there, but it was important for them. It seems all parents want their children to have a better life than they had growing up and mine were no different.

What my parents could not possibly understand was how lonely and out of place I was at that school. I felt so very different from my peers and was unable to verbalize or even comprehend what was going on inside me. My family did not practice their religion in the same strict manner as I was being taught at the school, and I was the youngest and only fat child in my class. I had no coping skills as to how to deal with my discomfort. I know that I used food as an escape from my surroundings and to comfort me. Food had also become my "best friend" at a very young age and very often it seemed that it was my only refuge. I firmly believe that my food addiction may have already begun by this time and most likely just got more firmly established during those formative years.

In a writing class I took a few years ago, we were asked to write about a vivid childhood memory, as if we were living it. I could think of quite a few, but one memory stood out in my mind. Let me share with you a memorable day from my confusing and painful childhood, where my self-constructed prison of fat and isolation began to develop and embody itself deep within my soul. This story will offer you a glimpse of my inner world when I was that fat eight and a half year-old child.

I walk down my street careful to keep myself small and unnoticed. I reach the end of the street and enter our local corner store. As I get closer, I fantasize about all the glorious things I will soon see. I dream about just how much candy the money I bring will buy for me. I can feel my eyes tear up with anticipation and I can almost feel all the stuff. It seems so vivid. I see just so many different sizes, shapes and beautiful colors. My tongue first gets dry and then my saliva starts to flow and I can imagine the bold tastes, some sweet, some salty, some sticky, some dry and still others hot and spicy. Some are so sweet, they make my teeth hurt and others stick to my teeth and need my tongue to work hard at pulling it away from the holes in my teeth and giving me the full impact of how crunchy and gooey it is. I am so excited; I can barely stand the "endless walk" of three blocks. There it is; I can see the store. Here is the glorious kingdom of "penny candy" and I have money and can get some. I think about what I want and already my mind goes into a blur. I want it all! I think if only I could just have as much as I want all the time. Maybe one day I'll have my own store filled with treats and lots of stuff I could have whenever I want. No one telling me to share with my brothers or that I have had enough.

I enter the store and head straight over to the candy counter as in a dream. I am finally here. Oh my, just look at all those pretty colors. I imagine what they will taste like when they squish around in my mouth. My mind becomes a whir as I start to remember the last time I had each type. Do I want the same ones I had when I went to my uncles last week or do I want to try something different? If I do, what if it does not taste good and I wasted my money? If I get some and don't enjoy it, when can I come back again for more? How will I hide it so mom does not see it all?

I take my mind away from this, because it makes me feel bad and it is not important now. Now I must decide what I want before Hymie comes over. I wonder just how much I can buy with the coin I took out of my mother's "special" place in her bedroom drawer. I have kept it hidden in my pocket and will give it to Hymie and he can tell me how much candy I get to pick. My mother called it a "Silver Dollar" like it was something important, but she had so many, I'm sure she will never notice that a few are missing, will she? What I do know is that Hymie did not seem to mind when I handed it to him the last time. As a matter of fact, he looked at it almost too closely, then lifted up one of his eyes to look at me and then gave me an odd smile, where the corner of the left side of his mouth slightly tipped upward while he stared directly at me. Today he seems almost excited to see me.

I feel myself getting more excited and almost feel like I can barely speak. My mouth is so dry and I think I need a soda, but I don't want to waste my money on that. As I gaze at the candy in boxes I start to imagine the sticky sweetness of the Raisinets – one of my favorites. I am thinking about the crunchy candy with nuts and caramel. Sometimes those make my teeth scream, but it is not that bad. I love the chocolate ones like M&M's but then I also like the fireballs and rock candy. Oh yeah, then there's Pez candy – those make me giggle and I love playing with the pop top, that is just so fun. I like to have the wax ones after I eat the "Pick up stick" powder candy because these burn my tongue and the liquid wets my mouth, mixes with the dry powder and then it all slides down my throat and ends up in my stomach. I want to get some gum, but the last time the teacher stuck me in the corner and told me if I did it again, I would end up at the principal's office. That makes me scared. What should I do? Maybe, I will just get a pack of Beeman's and just not chew it in class. Yeah, that's what I'll do.

Oh, here he comes; I better hurry up and decide before he asks me. I don't like it when he yells at me to hurry. It makes me forget what I wanted. This is just so exciting; I can feel my insides fluttering and my mouth watering. I hope I can wait till later and not eat it all up now. I want to bring some to school tomorrow.

Hymie stands behind the counter and I point out what I want. He is putting them in a bag and I can see the brown bag start to puff out and get heavier. It's all mine, wow! They call it penny candy, but some cost more; like the long thick pretzels I like so much cost 3 cents each. If I get too many that will use up all my money too fast, so I better only get two of them? But, I love how they crunch when I stuff them in my mouth. Maybe I better get three?

And I have to remember to get those red licorice whips because they last a real long time and I forgot to get them the last time. I like to carry them in my pockets, because they do not leak or stick and make a mess like chocolate. It's important to always have some candy wherever I go.

I leave the store and decide to eat my Raisinets now and then I will have my gum later. I will get a push-up rocket when the ice cream truck comes and save the rest of the candy for school. Boy, that silver dollar sure buys a lot of stuff. This bag is so full. I start to wonder just how I'll bring the bag of candy to school and eat it without anyone asking me for any. I hate it when they want my candy. It is mine, I bought it and it's all mine. Besides those kids are always so mean to me and only act nice to me when I have candy or something they want. Let them buy their own candy if they want some.

The next day I hide my stash in my schoolbag and go outside till the bus comes. I keep thinking about what I wish I could eat now, but I can't let anyone see me. When the bus comes, I go up the steps and look for a seat where I can be alone. I can already hear some of them saying mean things about me and stumble down to the back of the bus. Most of them won't let me sit next to them, not that I would want to anyway. I take a seat near the back all by myself while I act like I don't care. That's the hardest part, even more than their making fun of me and calling me fatty pants. Sometimes, it hurts so bad I just want to cry, but as soon as I feel my eyes getting wet, I have to stop myself so they don't see. Sometimes, I wish I could just throw something hard at them and make them stop and just leave me alone. I am so afraid, if I did, they would just hurt me.

The bus driver tells everyone to settle down and stay in their seats. Thank God, now they will forget about me and leave me alone. I hate taking the bus to school; I wish mom would just drive me.

I can see the school coming up on the right. I decide to wait till everyone else gets off and I slowly step off the bus and walk towards the front door of the school. I am getting excited about when I can open up my bag of candy and have some without anyone noticing me.

I go up the stairs, turn left, go down two hallways and turn into Rabbi Shiner's classroom and take my seat. I watch to see if anyone is around looking at me and stick my hand into my blue schoolbag and quickly take out my candy and stick it into my desk. I am pretty sure no one saw me. They all seem busy laughing and talking to each other. Good, I slowly reach into my desk, pull out a fireball and try to unwrap it without making any noise. I put the glowing red ball in my mouth already expecting what it will be like. As I suck on the hard sweet ball, I feel sparks flashing on my tongue and then it rolls around my mouth making my cheeks pucker with sweet explosions.

So, who cares if those kids don't like me, I don't need them anyway. They are not so special. I am the one with the candy, not them. As I finish up chewing the last of it, I decide now I want some chocolate. I secretly slide my hand into my bag again and feel for a Krackle chocolate. I love these. It is like eating Rice Krispies covered in chocolate. Yum!! Oh no, Rabbi Shiner is watching me. I don't think he actually saw me eating, did he? We are not supposed to chew gum or eat anything in class. That is such a stupid rule and who made it up anyway?

Is he talking to me? What did he say? I think he asked if I was chewing anything. Should I lie? I don't want him to make fun of me in front of everyone. I don't want to get into trouble. It would really make my parents upset. Oh no, he is coming over here. What is he going to do to me? He is opening up my desk and he found my bag. Now, he is opening it and looking inside. I better listen to what he is saying to me.

"Shayna did you bring this entire bag of candy to school for yourself?"

It feels like I swallowed my tongue, but I hear myself say: "I wanted some for recess and lunch." I try hard not to look directly at him; afraid I may break down and cry.

"You know I told you not to eat anything in class, don't you?"

I can feel his eyes on me like pointed darts. My eyes begin to fill with water, but I hold it in and am determined not to cry. Then all the kids will really laugh at me. I think to myself, I wish I could run away forever. I end up saying: "I was hungry and I only had one piece."

He stares at me as if he can see through my brain and hear what I am thinking and he says: "If you want to pass it around and share with the entire class, then I'll make an exception and everyone will have a special treat today."

The first thought that comes to me is: "What, I can't believe he'd ask me to give away any of my candy. It's mine and I paid for it. It is not theirs and I won't give them any! Why should I. I hate them all anyway!"

He says louder now: "Shayna, are you going to share it or do I have to take it away from you?

I surprise myself and say out loud: "NO. It's mine. They can't have any."

He looks so surprised and then after a moment shakes his head gives me a sad look and says: "That's too bad. I'm sorry you feel that way." He takes away my bag of penny candy and puts it on the top of his desk at the front of the room.

I can barely sit still. How can he do that to me? It's just not fair. Who does he think he is? He's not my parents. I want my candy back! I can feel my body shaking. I almost feel like one of those rabid dogs I saw on TV. I am just so mad. He had no right to take my stuff away from me. I want to yell at him, but that would get me into trouble for sure.

I hate it here with all their stupid rules. I am so filled with rage that it takes a while for me to remember I am inside a classroom with other kids. As I come out of my angry haze I begin to notice that all the kids are just staring at me. I can feel myself shrinking inside and feeling such hate and despair. I wonder if they will be mad at me for not giving them some of my candy or if they just don't care. They don't like me anyway. I know they'll tease me at recess like they always do. Stupid kids, I want my candy back. I spend the rest of the day alone and seething with feelings of anger, frustration, embarrassment and anxiety. I plan how I can hide my candy better the next time."

Well, was this the kind of memory that you have from your childhood? I sure hope not. I am pretty sure that was the beginning of my feeling like an outsider and distancing myself and my "insides" from others. I can remember to this day, exactly how it felt. I was outside some invisible barrier looking in at everyone else while they all belonged to some kind of secret club that I was not a part of. As a budding food addict, just starting down the road to where food took a powerful place in my adapting and functioning in life, I can see how I was really like a square peg pushing to fit into a round hold and never quite being able to.

As I got a few years older, I remember so clearly how my mother and my relatives would often say to me: "Susan, you have such a pretty face, if only you could lose some weight." Even at the young age of around ten, I knew my fat was a prison and that it would only get worse as I got older, but I did not know how to get out. The saddest part is that I knew no other way. My "sweets" gave my life a measure of pleasure and joy and seemed to work at sedating me for a very long time.

Remembering this gives me such sadness for that little girl, who knew no better, but had already learned her way of adapting and surviving in the difficult years of childhood. Everyone finds their own coping mechanism, but for me, food was a dysfunctional one at best.

So, maybe now you can understand, how being fat from fourth grade on and already being so hung up on sweets, just how excited and grateful I am today for having found my solutions of FA, (Food Addicts In Recovery) and "The Weight Loss Cure" Protocol. Now I can actually have a thin body and not be struggling every waking moment with the need for flour and sugar products. That was such a living hell that I felt stuck in for such a large portion of my life. I pray every day with all the strength that I possess inside of me that it is finally behind me.

If any of my childhood feelings or experiences ring true for you or someone close to you, do yourself a favor and check out FA and "The Weight Loss Cure." Feel free to send me an e-mail if I can be of any help to you.

You can reach me at FatNoMoreBook@gmail.com.

My main mission in this lifetime is to help someone else by using my experience, strength, and hope. I want to help keep others from going through any of the pain that I lived with for such a long time.

If you can't stop thinking about food, obsessing about food, constantly reading cookbooks, unable to stop at a few cookies or candies or snack foods, feel that your life is "run by food", are anorexic, bulimic, a binger, or just fat and unable to stop eating long enough to lose the excess weight, you may be a food addict.

CHAPTER 3

To the Struggling Food Addict

If you can't stop thinking about food, obsessing about food, constantly reading cookbooks, unable to stop at a few cookies or candies or snack foods, feel that your life is "run by food", are anorexic, bulimic, a binger, or just fat and unable to stop eating long enough to lose the excess weight, you may be a food addict. I know that you may consider this possibility to be a "hard pill to swallow", and that it might be quite humbling for you, but at least consider it and know that if you identify at all, then there is a solution for you.

At one time, I had thought that I had read every self-help and diet book and tried almost every diet, weight loss program, or suggested "way to live", that was available out there, but the only program that ever truly gave me a "living solution" was FA, Food Addicts in Recovery.

If you even think you may have a serious, unsolvable problem with food, I strongly suggest you check out their web site, www.foodaddicts.org and attend some of their meetings. It will not hurt for you to check them out and you really have nothing to lose. You may even find yourself surprised that the program speaks to you, and offers you an understanding of things that you have struggled with for years.

I can honestly say FA saved my life, my sanity, and my marriage. My food addiction had made me so very unhappy. At times I felt I could barely go on, and my life took so much effort every day. FA and the 12 Step Program of recovery helped take away my obsession and food cravings and allowed me to live a life of freedom and neutrality around food. It also gave me the side benefit of a feeling of inner peace and serenity.

Now that I have said that crucial fact, I want to add that even though my food addiction was finally resolved and I was "in recovery" where I no longer craved food or was obsessed with food, that I had been plagued with for as long as I can remember, I reached a point where I still had fat to lose and no matter what I did it would not come off. It was explained to me by a few doctors that it was due to reaching what is called my personal "Set Point".

Once that happened, I also coincidentally and simultaneously entered the dreaded "Perimenopause" phase of my womanhood cycle and I began to gain weight with what seemed like no end point in sight. My female body seemed to blow up like a balloon with loss of my shape. I went to my doctors but they were unable to find any definitive answer or valid reason for what my body was going through.

What they did tell me was that all my years of yo-yo dieting had caught up with me and I would have to "accept myself fat" and "grin and bear it". I was told to "Just accept it is the body weight your body seems to want."

I just could NOT accept what I judged as their insensitive retorts. Being the determined woman that I am, although it got me down for a while and I became somewhat depressed, I never allowed myself to completely give up my hope to be thin. I felt like there was this slim woman trapped inside of my fat body who was struggling to be let out and thrive. Then after much heartache and struggle, one day, I found the "Weight Loss Cure".

I read this book from cover to cover and read the entire scientific paper written by Dr. Simeone, and for once all the pieces of the puzzle and answers I had been looking for were right there. This amazing doctor understood it all and wrote in his paper that he could help people like me. Maybe, finally I would get my help.

If anything that I have said sounds familiar or the least bit interesting at all to you, then KEEP READING!!

Remember there is ALWAYS hope. So don't you give up yet, either!!

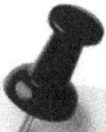

According to the medical weight charts, I was still 10-15 pounds above the accepted normal "healthy weight", but no matter how little I ate, what type of food was added, or what food plan I was put on, I could not get the excess weight off.

CHAPTER 4

My Personal Experience with Joining FA, Food Addicts in Recovery

After about 18 years in OA, Overeater's Anonymous, a 12 Step program of recovery for "Compulsive Overeaters", I went through a very difficult and painful period of my life. I was running a busy dental practice with all the stresses and challenges that go along with direct patient care, in addition to running a business and trying to do it all well. I had become complacent with my OA program and what I had been doing for many years and I found myself making excuses and justifying ways to change my planned way of eating. I stopped being honest with myself, my support group and fellowship and I began to slip and slide and make poor food choices for myself. I told myself that I could eat like everyone else in the world and have a little extra here and there as I wanted. I even told myself that occasionally I could eat sugar-free snack type foods if they were low calorie or dietetic.

Basically, I had become quite frustrated after being in OA for so many years and still having more weight to lose. I decided I needed more than what OA offered me and I sought help from a Bariatrician, a doctor specializing in weight loss. I told him I needed help to lose my last 30 or so pounds and asked that he put me on the Fen-Phen, (Fenfluramine-Phentermine) diet plan. He told me I was a good candidate, gave me some instruction and education on what I was going to do, dispensed the medications and I started on the plan. I followed his basic diet plan and also chose not to eat anything with sugar or flour, as I had learned in OA. On this drug regimen and diet plan, I was finally able to be successful in losing all my remaining excess weight.

However, once my weight was off, I did not want to keep taking diet pills and I hated the feeling of always feeling "spacey", dry mouthed and euphoric. I had also become bored with his diet and specific way of eating my meals and I wanted more food choices, especially since I felt so thin and powerful.

That thought process led to my fall from my success with Fen-Phen. It started so innocently by my choosing to have grapes after dinnertime as a snack before bedtime. If I didn't want it then, I told myself, I could have it later at night should I wake up, which I occasionally did. What began to happen was that I would get up at night, feel hungry and eat my grapes and within a short period of time, I started getting up at night just to eat my grapes.

Then my old behavior of "sleep-eating" reared its ugly head again. I used to do this a lot before I joined OA and had truly believed that it was over and in the past. I would get up in the middle of the night drowsy from sleep, go down to the kitchen, eat something out of the refrigerator, and then go back up to bed. When I woke up the next morning, I barely remembered going to the kitchen and eating in the middle of the night.

Shortly thereafter, other old behaviors began to slip back into my life. For example, I noticed myself hiding food around the house, sneaking around trying to eat extra and lying to my husband, so he wouldn't know what I was doing with food. Since I had always considered myself a "Compulsive Overeater", as defined in OA, and hadn't yet realized that I was actually a "food addict", I began to eat more and more snack type foods and then eat them in large quantities. I ate diet popsicles, diet fudgsicles, diet hot chocolate, diet candy, diet Jell-O, non-sugared frozen yogurt and many types of 'health foods'. Before I realized it, I was craving all my old binge foods again and feeling obsessed with food day and night. In time I figured out that I had been changing my boundaries around food to fit my whims until I eventually had no boundaries at all.

I think I realized on some deeper level that I had to be more than just a "compulsive overeater", because I saw that once I started eating these foods, I was craving them constantly and could NOT stop myself. I would feel so badly about what I was doing with food including all the hiding, sneaking around and lying about it to everyone. I felt constant shame and guilt and fear around the food once again.

My many years in OA, had taught me that this was not normal or healthy behavior, so I felt like an OA failure. I had told myself and many others for so many years that I was a success in OA, since I had not eaten anything with sugar or flour for a very long time. In truth, however, I had had periods of "slipping" with eating large quantities of proteins and vegetables, eating more than what was on my food plan and long periods of struggling and "white knuckling". Although I was told the goal was to have a serene, peaceful and consistent *Abstinence*** with food, I could not seem to achieve that serenity or to reach my goal weight.

After stopping the Fen-Phen diet and going back to my old ways of eating, I soon started eating sugar and flour products

---

** **In FA, Abstinence is defined as weighing, measuring and committing one's food to a qualified sponsor in the program, and abstaining from all refined carbohydrates and sugars.**

and within a short period of time I had not only gained back the weight I lost from Fen-Phen, but I also regained most of the weight I had lost over the years in OA. I returned to going out and eating at fast food restaurants, bakeries, and binging on whatever I wanted. I became so miserable, hopeless and even more depressed than ever before. None of my clothes fit and I didn't want to leave the house. I just wanted to hide from the world and die from shame!

Well, it seems the old adage: "It's darkest before the dawn" was true for me. I was crying in my husband's arms one night in our home in front of our fireplace, when I just cried out: "I am an addict with food". At that moment it was so very clear to me and I knew it in my core and in every cell of my body from my head to my toe. I didn't know if there was a solution to my problem, but I knew I was licked. My husband suggested I find an OA meeting and try again. I was desperate and willing to do so, but to be honest I had very little hope that anything I found out there could work for me. How wrong I was!

I went to a few different meetings and to my absolute amazement, I found a meeting that had been OA, but had just changed to become FA only 6 weeks earlier. FA, Food Addicts in Recovery Anonymous, is a 12 Step, spiritual program, based on the same foundation and principles of AA, Alcoholics Anonymous.

What I noticed at this new FA meeting was that everyone seemed happy and most of them were thin. When they shared, they said very positive things and spoke about hope and how FA had completely changed their lives for the better. I was intrigued and began to wish I could feel the way they did. They suggested going to a few meetings and deciding if it was right for me, and if so to get a sponsor to help guide me through the program. I already knew from my many years in OA, that I would need a sponsor in order to have any success at all.

So with fear and much doubt, I found a sponsor to help guide and teach me the program and within a couple of weeks to my utter amazement, I found myself becoming free from the cravings and obsessions with food, and gaining a feeling of serenity. I was delighted that I had found an Abstinence that I hadn't experienced in many years and thought would never be possible for me again. I followed all the suggestions given to me by my sponsor and other successful members of FA and found my weight slowly coming off again and my depression and hopelessness lifting. It definitely helped me with my food addiction and in changing my life for the better.

However, although FA was my salvation and the answer to stop my food addiction and was very important for me in many respects, it still was not the answer for me to lose all my excess weight.

I am now going to share a little more, in depth, about my experience in FA. I joined FA in August of 1998 and grew to love my FA Twelve Step program dearly. I felt at the time that it literally saved my life. I no longer woke up each and every day discouraged and wanting to die. I no longer felt obsessed and compelled to eat all the time, even when I was not hungry. The compulsion to eat and binge until I was ill was gone. Food became somewhat neutral for me and in time I found an inner serenity and peacefulness that I had never experienced before.

I was told by my sponsor and many other FA members that in time my body would rid itself of all the extra pounds and normalize itself, that I would be thin, healthy and no longer be hungry except when it came to my mealtimes. This was one of the many promises those before me told me to expect if I followed their example. I had met so many people attesting to this fact, that I believed it would also be true for me.

The truth is that many of their promises of how I could live my life without the addiction to food did actually materialize for me. However, as I wrote earlier, from the beginning my weight came off very, very slowly, much slower than others in FA, including my sponsor, was used to seeing. Where others lost ten pounds the first month, I lost five pounds. Where others lost all their weight within a few months to one year with an average weight loss of 25 to 100 pounds, I only lost 35 pounds the first year and it took another year of trying various food plans to lose another 18 pounds, and it was still not a stable weight. My weight would just keep creeping up. I could never reach the point where my doctors and the weight charts said was "normal" for my height and body type.

According to the medical weight charts, I was still 10-15 pounds above the accepted normal "healthy weight", but no matter how little I ate, what type of food was added, or what food plan I was put on, I could not get the excess weight off. This excess fat was on my abdomen, thighs, hips, buttocks, and upper inner arms. My inner thighs also had loose flesh and I had stretch marks all over my body from childhood obesity.

I was actually so delighted to be thinner, that I would have been willing to accept this state for the rest of my life, if it wasn't for the fact that my weight would just not stabilize. I would have been happy to keep following my food plan, even though it was very strict, extremely limited and only 1000 calories/day. There was also a lot of concern that this plan was a lot less calories than my primary care doctor and my nutritionist told me I needed to eat in order to "maintain my normal daily functions".

I was told that most FA'ers on my food plan kept losing weight and food had to be added back into their food plan in order to give back the necessary calories their bodies needed to be healthy and maintain their daily metabolic needs. I was told that my food plan, which had minimal grain and minimal fat, was not healthy for the long term. Supposedly, it would lead to problems for me over time.

Well once again I felt, as the expression goes, like I was "between a rock and a hard place". My body was NOT responding like everyone else's. Again!! I was heavier than my peers and seemed to be slowly gaining the weight back that I had lost. This was like Déjà Vu to me; for as I wrote earlier, I was fully aware that my metabolism had never responded like everyone else's, starting from the time I was a pre-teenager and got obese between the ages of eight to ten. I felt like I lived in a kind of "twilight zone" and it was all so crazy making for me.

It made me begin to doubt myself again and really made me feel different from almost everyone else. Very few people I spoke to in the FA Program seemed to be able to understand. Their food plans worked for them. I began to doubt my reality and I even asked myself: "Was I cheating? Was I eating extra calories without my awareness? Was I being taken over by a "Body Snatcher", when I wasn't aware of it?" My answer was NO!! What hurt me the most was the response I received from most of my peers and mentors in FA when they began to question my honesty and my commitment.

I knew I was not cheating and yet I started to wonder if I was somehow "blocking out" eating. Could I be eating food and simply "forgetting", but I knew I was not. I felt so frustrated and knew that I just could not give up. I finally had the food cravings, the obsession and the compulsion removed, and that was a miracle that I planned on keeping. I couldn't leave FA, but I knew that I needed something more, when my peers and my own FA recovery group doubted me. I felt abandoned and betrayed by them. They did not understand, just like all the doctors I had seen. It then became very clear to me that this group could no longer be my main support system and once again I felt all alone!

Adding to my frustration, my sponsor at the time had just entered Menopause and had developed a thyroid condition, whereby she herself had gained a lot of weight. She was struggling herself and trying to also help me. Ultimately, she got frustrated and told me that she needed to take care of herself and I had to find a new sponsor. After all my years of struggling with weight and food addiction, and especially my recovery time in FA, I had learned that I could not deal with this by myself. Truly, no one on this earth should really have to go it all alone. I am convinced that we all need others to share their experience, strength and hope with us from time to time. I believe this is especially true for food addicts in recovery.

So there I was with over five years of clean Abstinence in FA and I was struggling to maintain my 125 pound body weight. I had begun to regain some of my lost weight and was feeling very dismayed. I had changed nothing of any significance and was still following all the same disciplines. I was still exercising on my treadmill 30 minutes a day and following my simple, basic 1000 calorie food plan.

I ended up gaining a total of 27 pounds in the next 1 and ½ to 2 years, without any reprieve in sight. Nothing I tried stopped my weight gain! I actually felt like that powerless, fat, little kid all over again. It was terrible. I went to everyone I could think of for help, but no one could! I had even lost a lot of my energy, was tired a lot and I did not feel like doing very much most days. All my blood tests were normal and yet I had gained 27 pounds with no understandable or logical reason.

I became despondent, depressed, and resigned to being obese once again. I seemed to be completely powerless over the changes going on in my body. This "personal torment', I write about, went on for about 2 and ½ years, before I heard about the book, "The Weight Loss Cure".

I had gotten a new sponsor who was willing to listen to my despair, offer suggestions if she had any, and be available to me as a loving resource that kept me staying committed and following my 12 Step FA program. She was one of the wonderful people that had heard about the book;" The Weight Loss Cure" and mentioned it to me as something I might want to check out. To this day I remain very grateful to her for offering me something I might never have found on my own.

This book was my first ray of hope, since my finding FA recovery in 1998. Everyone needs to have some hope to truly live! In this book, Kevin Trudeau wrote about a doctor in a clinic in Argentina, Dr. Simeone, who had a working theory about excess weight and a solution about how to get thin. I was ready to try anything. At that point I felt that I would even go to Argentina and be checked into his HCG clinic. I had already tried every potion, pill, doctor's suggestion, and gimmick that had made any sense to me, but nothing had gotten my excess weight off. I decided that I had to find out more and I tracked down and read Dr. Simeone's manuscript.

After reading it, I felt totally understood. My problem was explained in a way that made sense to me. This doctor said there was a CURE, not just a possibility to lose weight, but a real cure. I felt real hope returning for the first time in many, many years. Dr. Simeone seemed to tell "my story", starting from my childhood obesity all the way to the present day weight dilemma.

My reaction to his manuscript was one of relief and excitement. I decided then and there to pursue the possibility and follow his plan if it was appropriate for me. This doctor confirmed that I was not just a "fat, lazy slob" eating "unknowingly", and I could let go of those harsh judgments I thought about myself. I was actually a woman with an "out-of-balance hypothalamus" causing my obesity, lack of energy and ongoing feelings of depression.

You see, when I started my FA food plan in 1998, one thing that never changed that I was told would change, was my true hunger level. (Note, of course that when the food plan is fewer calories than the bodies' metabolic index tests say you need daily, it is no wonder I was hungry). As I already mentioned, I had been told by those FA'ers before me that my body would eventually become normalized and stable, reach its "ideal, slim, healthy weight" and I would only be truly hungry at my three planned meals.

For my first 7 years in FA following my food plan, I would eat 3 weighed and measured, bulky meals and would then feel "stuffed" and uncomfortable. The food plan that my counterparts and I were given were intended to offer lots of vegetables in order to give us enough bulk to feel satisfied and fulfill our hunger without adding up to lots of calories. However, for me the bulky salad and cooked vegetables seemed to just "sit" stuffed into my stomach. I was also hungry a lot of the time during the day and night. It did not feel like cravings or "false hunger". I knew after a while and believe now, that it was not emotional hunger. I was feeling actual hunger. I was hypoglycemic and not getting the interim small snacks of healthy food that I needed.

One time I had tried eating 6 small meals as an experiment, suggested by one of my FA sponsors, and it actually helped my hunger. Those stuffed feelings that I would experience after each large meal was gone and I was less hungry during the day, but my hunger was never fully eliminated. When I was told to add more calories into my daily plan for my health, my weight crept up again, but I did feel better. (Note-I was eating an average of 1200 calories a day.) However, no matter what amount of calories I ate, be it 900, 1000 or 1200 calories, all of my excess weight did not come off, and continued over time to increase.

It was all so confusing to me. I had read in many medical and diet books that in order to maintain one's weight, "calories in should equal calories out". That meant that I needed to eat less to lose the extra weight and if my BMI was 1250, I should at the least be maintaining my weight and not gaining. However, my reality was that no matter what I did, my weight did not budge; not even when I reduced my calories to 800/day. I was also told that I should exercise more, but I had lost the desire to exercise since I had so little energy and felt so tired all the time.

It seemed that the supposed "rules" did not work for me. It made me feel different and somehow "defective". I felt I couldn't get any medical help since most of the doctors did not believe me. How unfair and isolating that was for me! What a way to live. I definitely was not living a full, joyful life. It seemed that I was only surviving one day at a time and desperately seeking ways to cope and retain some hope and purpose in my life.

I know some might say: "Just get over it. Accept yourself being larger and move on!" I think this could work for many people, but for me, being an active and fully committed member of FA, where one's peers watch you very closely, it was NOT acceptable to me. Also, I was still so emotionally affected from my childhood obesity, that I felt I had to get thin, for me to fully recover the "emotional losses" and get past my childhood issues.

So, you can only imagine just how delighted and hopeful I was after finding the "Weight Loss Cure" and being able to use it as my ultimate stepping stone to finally getting my excess weight off.

CHAPTER 5

My Reflections on Obesity and Finding HCG

Obesity is an illness that is disfiguring and debilitating. Being an obese person has caused me a lot of shame, humiliation, and feeling different from my peers. I remember that when I was young and in gym class, I had to wear a different uniform, since the school uniform was not made in my size. I would always need to be hyper aware of what I looked like and then act a certain way, so that my peers would not judge me too harshly or bully me. It was especially stressful for me when I wore shorts and had to go out in public. Being obese as a teen and young adult limited my functioning socially around both boys and girls alike. Girls would usually feel superior to me and treat me as if I were lazy and had no willpower, while most boys acted uninterested or disgusted, depending on how fat I was at the time.

I have always felt that I had to act better and be better in general just to be in the same "game", but no matter what I did, I still could never measure up. The constant bombardment in magazines and on television showing the "ideal American woman", and describing fat women as "having issues", being pitied and being unacceptable, led to my feeling much shame and humiliation. It is a common fact and understood by most people, that being thin will get you further in life and give you more power over others.

Here is a quote taken from the book:" Rethinking Thin" by Gina Kolata; "Life as a fat person can be hard and societies judgment harsh. Studies have found that fat people are less likely to get admitted to elite colleges, less likely to be hired for a job, make less money when they are hired, and are less likely to be promoted."

This disease of obesity is still so misunderstood by everyone including the medical profession. They come up with the current philosophy of the day that is determined from what seems to fit the majority of people. We are all told that our body weight is determined by the equation; food in and energy out equals our final weight. However, doctors know that this is not the complete answer. They know it does not explain many of their patient's weight and metabolism issues. This equation does not account for those times when one patient gains weight on the exact same food plan as another patient of the same height and weight and activity level.

Yet when questioned directly, most doctors will act like they know all the answers; even if today's "truth" ends up being tomorrow's "misdiagnosis". History has proven that in time the lack of information during one decade becomes replaced in the next decade with a newer theory from either new medical knowledge, or a kind of "recycled' thinking using a new paradigm.

The problem with obesity as an illness is the judgments that society in general makes on obese people. It is commonly assumed that larger people must be eating in private and getting fat due to overeating and cheating. Although this is true for many heavy people, who do overeat in private, it does NOT account for everyone that has weight issues.

This judgment can become extremely traumatizing, as I found out from my own experience following my 12 Step food addiction program. The majority of people in my FA program were able to lose and maintain their goal weight without too much trouble. However, there were some of us that had the additional burden of either a medical problem or a "metabolic obesity disease", where we either never lost all our excess fat or lost and regained it no matter how little we ate. This often led to our own peer groups judging us, assuming we were cheating and lying. It created for me what I call a "crazy making" position that became very precarious for me. What I learned the hard way is that there are just too many naïve people out there, who assume and act like they know it all and in reality, they do not.

I was determined to find a solution to my excess weight problem and also to help others I knew, that had been obese and lost weight, but was still unable to get all their weight off and keep it off. I wanted success for all of us.

When I first read Kevin's book and felt hope, I started wondering just how I could follow it. At first, I thought the simplest way was to check myself into a clinic and have them do it all for me. It would mean my having to take off more than one month from my "normal life" and get full coverage at my business. I was very concerned about my business and the financial stresses, my being away would create. I felt strongly, however, that this could give me my lifetime dream and a promise of a real cure, and I could not miss the opportunity.

Although I felt ready and willing to do whatever it took to attain my dream, I wanted to exhaust any possibility of going to a local clinic or at least one within the USA. As I searched for available clinics I could find nothing locally and none within the USA that had in-patient treatment. I remember feeling so angry and disillusioned, but my "fighter" instinct stepped in and I decided to reread everything in Kevin's book on the initial Phase 1 protocol. I decided that I could start my process of "getting healthier" by following Phase 1 while I figured out what the options were for Phase 2.

After two weeks of using the recommended cleanses and having two colonics, I began to feel better physically and my optimistic attitude returned. Getting a little hope back actually gave my life purpose and direction again. I decided I would follow the book, get "cured", attain my dream to be thin and look normal, and then write my own book to help others. Sharing it with others also going through my pain was now my goal. Somehow, I truly believed it would work. My longtime goal and vision had always been to help others be happier, gain self-esteem and reach their goals, and now I was on my way again.

As I continued to research the information in Kevin's book, I was given web sites to go to for further information. In one of the web sites discussing "The Cure", I read a comment that "not everyone" was accepted for the treatment. That possible rejection gave me a lot of anxiety and fear. Would I be refused and not be allowed to even try it?

I called some of the suggested clinics and left messages of my interest. However, only one clinic in the USA returned my call, HCG Medical. I told them my current status, my past history, answered all their questions and discussed what I was looking for. The representative told me they would speak to their medical director and get back to me. I asked many questions about the process and was told that they had people following the protocol at home, giving themselves the required daily injections and having incredible success. I must admit, the idea of giving myself injections really freaked me out at first, but I decided to pursue it anyway. I told myself that if I was accepted, I could "act as if" I could do it. This mindset and way of thinking allowed me to keep moving forward and not give up.

About 1 week later, the representative from HCG Medical called me back and told me they were sending me an e-mail with a lab slip for the pre-requisite blood tests and their medical history forms that I needed to fill out and send back to them; which I did. The process took 3 more weeks. During that time I felt like I was on "pins and needles", just waiting to hear if I was a good candidate for "the Protocol". When I got the call from HCG Medical telling me I was approved and they would call in the prescription to start the HCG, I actually felt like I had won the lottery. At least now I had a chance.

I had so many questions, as I always do, and all of the members of the staff at HCG Medical were wonderful! Whenever I spoke with someone they were always encouraging, helpful and able to offer support and inspiration to me. Not only were they always gracious and willing to answer my questions when I started the "Weight Loss Cure" process, but they were also always willing to guide me. They took time to help me understand the suggestions that occasionally baffled me, helped me order any needed supplies and were extremely helpful when I did not lose all the weight I wanted to during the first go around, and helped me with the protocol a second time.

Their incredible personal service and concern for my welfare made me wish that all medical and doctor's offices had the same personality skills and customer service that the staff of HCG offered. I am so very grateful for all they did for me.

I had finally found the solution that I wanted for myself and others like me. Obesity can be a distant memory of yours and not distort your body or your life any more. You might even be able to start your process earlier than I did and prevent yourself from ever becoming really obese in the first place. You may never have to find out what the public's prejudice is like when one is obese.

CHAPTER 6

In Summary
What I Have Learned

Being a fat child felt like a kind of "torture" for me; the slow and steady kind.

Generally speaking, most Caretakers give food to show love, and as we can all imagine, food can make a lonely child feel cared about. For so many of us, eating sugar and flour products can block out the pain of having poor social skills and fear of others. It keeps us occupied while others are socializing, it feels comforting going down, and somehow affords us a feeling of belonging.

Parents need to help guide their children and train them in effective socializing with others. Without any socializing skills to help a child grow thru the "trials of childhood", a child is left with no resources except using food or some other "relief seeking" replacement. Very often, the first thing a child is drawn to is food and sweets, and many times that is where they stop.

What happens when a child gets fat? Usually the caretakers try to stop the "snacks", but this can leave the child with feeling unloved and somehow "bad". This can be very confusing for a child. If they are left without any resources to deal with it, most will turn to some childish way to regain the lost love or to gain the attention from others. This can show up in many ways and sometimes in unhealthy and dysfunctional ones.

Just look at the large numbers of young people NOT being able to accept themselves as they are and needing to find some sense of self and control. Many of them go looking for things or substances to fulfill them, while others become anorexic or bulimic.

When a child gets fat or engages in dysfunctional food behaviors, their peers may laugh or mock them and many will call the child names and bully them. This further lowers a child's self-esteem, increases the fear they have of their peers and leads them into hiding-out and secretive behaviors. The final result becomes increased isolation and an assortment of self-damaging responses.

I can attest to the fact that the experience of being a fat child and all that it entails, never really leaves a person. It actually leaves scars deeper and more powerful than those created by surgery. My surgical, skin scars are dimming and easily covered up with clothing, but not so with my emotional wounds. As an adult I still carry all those emotional and spiritual scars, which continue to haunt me and affect my adult life in seemingly subtle ways. I am supposed to be able to get over it, and although intellectually I understand and have been able to move on and live a reasonably happy adult life, my "lost or stolen childhood" never totally stops affecting me in many insidious ways.

I can still hear and feel the taunting and bullying that I experienced over 45 plus years ago. Those demeaning comments other kids made about me can still sting and cause me to question myself at times. Thoughts of thinking of myself as ugly, stupid, unworthy, weak and worthless are marks hidden in my soul. My long ago child's experience of not being able to "fit into the world", still remains and will occasionally surprise me when I least expect it.

For those of you with children, whom you probably love more than life itself, and want to give them a better life and much more than what you had, please keep them from becoming obese. Do this one thing and you will not only save them from all the bullying, demeaning, life-damaging consequences of being a bullied, obese child, but you will also be giving them the gift of self-esteem and acceptance.

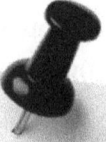

Eventually, it all came together like a puzzle and became easier to follow and almost rote for me, just like anything we do for a period of time.

CHAPTER 7

A Glimmer of Hope For Me

When I read Kevin Trudeau's book, for the first time in September of 2007, I was almost in tears. There was so much that made sense. I read that there were others just like me and they had found a cure. Then I read the testimonials on his web site and spoke personally with others that had followed Dr. Simeone's plan. It gave me my first "glimmer of hope". Could this be true? Could this really be my problem; what had been my albatross all these years, the prison that kept me feeling so different from others? What had kept me feeling so much self-pity about myself and my circumstances and the daily desperation, inner turmoil and pain! This desire to be like everyone else and feel "normal" had haunted me and driven me. It was my main focus and inner desire for so much of my life. I was so afraid to allow myself to feel any hope, but I did anyway.

    I tenaciously pursued this answer like I did everything else in my life, with 100% commitment. I read all I could about "The Cure'. I read the book over and over, again and again, and took copious notes until I understood it, believed it and was ready to follow it completely as it was written, no matter what it took. I was even ready to go to Germany, where Dr. Simeone treated patients or to his clinic in Argentina! Luckily and very gratefully, I did not have to leave the country to get my chance. As I mentioned earlier, I found HCG Medical in the United States, a terrific clinic with wonderful and kind people that helped me through the entire process, via the telephone.

Author's Personal Note:

  I used this "Weight Loss Cure" book as if it was a science text. I studied it seriously, reading and rereading the book and manuscript many times, taking copious notes, and reviewing it over and over until I truly understood it and knew in my heart and soul, that it was exactly right for me. I found that I had to return to my notes and the information constantly like a writer might use a dictionary or a religious person may use sacred scriptures with text references. There was just so very much to comprehend and figure out at first. Eventually, it all came together like a puzzle and became easier to follow and almost rote for me, just like anything we do for a period of time.

  The bottom line is I want to offer you this opportunity. Let me be the one who has done all the research for you and just be willing to believe what I have told you. Follow the path that I have suggested in this book, and I am sure that you will have the same amazing and wonderful results as I have had.

  To repeat a phrase from my 12 Step program: "YOU WILL BE AMAZED BEFORE YOU ARE HALFWAY THROUGH!"

CHAPTER 8

Deciding To Try "The Weight Loss Cure Program"

In early Sept.2007, my husband and I went on a vacation to Florida where I dedicated most of my time and energy to figuring out how I could start the Phase 1 plan. I wanted to give myself time to determine if the book would work for me and if I really wanted to follow it. I packed Kevin's book, Dr. Simeone's manuscript and the homeopathic cleanses that were suggested for Phase 1.

While on vacation, I took all the recommended supplements and cleanses and drank only spring water. I went walking daily for exercise and to get the suggested sunshine. I read all the literature and rigorously studied the diet. My plan was to read the book and decide if it was even possible for me to follow the strict regimen. As I read the book, a lot of feelings erupted within me. I felt such excitement and renewed hope that I had not felt for over four years. I could even feel an inner spark igniting within me.

Not surprising, I also felt fear that I would not be given the HCG treatment, or that if I did follow it, that it would not work for me. I had already been through so much and experienced so many diets, and all of them had failed me. What if this one failed me, too?

As I look back at it now, I think I had to believe it would work for me in order to meet my own emotional needs and to keep my sanity. As I have already shared, my desire was to find a solution and a cure for myself and then devote myself to helping others. I kept thinking about all the "lost souls" out there; my brothers and sisters that share my pain, my misery, and my loneliness in the "world of obesity".

I had always believed that my life's purpose was offering service to others from my own personal experiences and my overcoming of so many odds. My purpose had become clear to me during my years of treating phobic dental patients and in helping other suffering food addicts. However, I had lost much of my enthusiasm and that spark within when I gained almost 30 pounds while following my disciplined, 1000 calorie a day, FA food plan. During this eventful week in Florida, I began to notice that my inner spark and faith of my purpose was returning.

Dr. Simeone discussed a problematic, genetic tendency of being susceptible to getting obese. He explained quite well how a portion of our brain, called the Diencephalon, stores our "primitive animal instincts", and can "transfer pressure from one instinct to another". He wrote that a lonely and unhappy person, deprived of all emotional comfort and of all instant gratification, except the quieting of one's hunger and thirst, can use these outlets and turn to food for the pent up "instinct pressure", have it imbedded into the brain, and ultimately become obese. Yet, once this happens, no amount of psychotherapy or analysis, happiness, company of others, or gratification of other instincts will correct our condition. I could understand this by comparing it to a piece of paper being embossed. Once the embossing is imprinted onto the paper, it's always there, no matter what else is done or put onto the paper.

His explanation "told my tale" and summarized my life and what I had been living with for many years. I was a very lonely child who ate for comfort, the only outlet I had, and I became obese. My obesity led to my depression and a life I experienced as constantly yearning to be thin and being devoid of any joy. My own genetic tendency and my early childhood addiction to sugar and flour had been the start of my desperation and feelings of being different from others.

Many of you when you first read this may feel a sense of identification and possibly resignation and depression that you are stuck and there's no use in trying to fight your own genetics. It's very important for me to stop here for a moment and remind you, that I believe that there is a real solution for you; "The Weight Loss Cure" protocol.

Personally, my solution has been a combination of my Twelve Step FA program and the "Weight Loss Cure." Together, they have helped me get thin and allow me to continue to live a happy, productive and serene life.

Simeone's explanation of my weight issue told me that once the damage had occurred to my diencephalon and I became obese, diet alone could not cure it. My diencephalon became damaged when I was a very young child and what I needed was a way to correct it and to help it function more effectively.

There is a very important point I want to make here- In Dr. Simeone's manuscript, he says, "For a large body, more caloric energy is needed to heat it and the muscular effort to move an obese body is greater than a small body. This muscular effort consumes calories that must be provided by food". Thus, he goes on, "all factors being equal, a fat person require more food than a lean one". So, one would reason, that if a fat person eats only the additional food his body requires, he should be able to keep his weight stable. However, as all physicians that study this know, this is not true. Many obese patients actually gain weight on a diet that is calorically deficient for their basic needs. Therefore, there must be some other mechanism at work!"

This section of his manuscript rang so true to me from my own experience.

What about you?

As I wrote earlier, when my obesity began, I was a very young fourth grader and it was all so very confusing for me. I knew that I loved foods made with sugar and flour and that I felt very drawn to them. It seemed very strange to me, that I could get so fat so quickly, when I did not consume huge quantities of food. As I got a little older and more in tune with myself, I could accept that I ate too much, but even given that, the amount of calories eaten was very disproportionate to the amount of weight that I actually gained. When I went on a diet, I was never able to lose the expected amount or the proportionate amount in relation to what I had consumed.

When I read Dr. Simeone's manuscript, I was immediately struck by this man's full understanding of the obese patient's misery and effects of the disease. I was touched by his compassion and commitment towards this debilitating illness. He wrote on page 3 of his paper: "Persons suffering from this (obesity) disorder will get fat regardless of whether they eat excessively, normal, or less than normal."

This statement referred directly to me. My food intake and weight gain history was totally unexplainable. I would follow a strict FA food plan like others in my fellowship and I would gain weight while they would lose their excess weight. I would then cut back my calories and still I would continue to gain weight. I would strictly follow my nutritionist's weight loss food plan, and I would again gain weight. No one could understand why or give me any reasons for my gaining weight or keeping on the excess weight and it would make me feel very frustrated and somewhat "abnormal".

Many practitioners suggested that I had a higher set point than what the weight charts advised, and there was nothing I could do about it until a proven method to lower it was discovered. My nutritionist did a BMI test, showing that I needed 1250 calories per day, in order for me to maintain my body's normal, basic needs. However, when I ate 1250 calories a day, I would gain weight. My body just did NOT function the way they said it should.

When Dr. Simeone wrote the following, "It is not all about the calories", he was indeed referring to my metabolic status. That's why when I read it; I could feel my head nodding in agreement. On page 4, he wrote that "Thyroid medications do not touch these abnormal fat reserves." I did not know that and obviously most physicians don't either. I had always believed that the thyroid medication, that I took, would be the answer, but in fact, it is not the complete answer. My medicine gave my body some metabolic stasis, but did nothing for lowering my set point or ridding my body of its excess fat reserves.

Since I knew that my obesity began at such a young age, around 8 years old, I wondered if that's when my Hypothalamus and my Diencephalon got damaged. As I referred to earlier, my childhood was one of obesity and being ostracized by my peers; leading me to feeling different and becoming isolated and lonely. Ultimately I became extremely depressed and experienced my personal suffering and lack of joy.

The way I viewed it, there was my genetic tendency to obesity, my childhood sugar and flour addiction, the total lack of understanding from everyone around me and ultimately, my downward spiral and "demise." I know this may sound a little melodramatic, so let me describe this "demise" with the following childhood memories: I have many vivid memories of being called Chubby and having to shop at the Women's section of Lane Bryant when I was only 10 years old, being continuously told I had "baby fat' when I was in my late teens, feeling hungry often during the day and being told I was a pig, being called lazy when I felt weak and lethargic and unable to perform in sports like my peers, being constantly told: "You have such a pretty face, if only you would lose weight", developing "fat lady" stretch marks from the age of ten that were all over my body, and being unable to look like any other children my age, due to my distorted body shape.

If only someone knew Dr. Simeone's medical truth back then, that diet alone would not correct the damages done to my Diencephalon; perhaps my life could have been very different. Even now, at this present moment, medical science is still searching for the answers to this quandary. Maybe one day soon they will have more answers for us, but in the meantime, we have the "Weight Loss Cure" program.

Perhaps, dear readers, if you are willing to jump right in and follow what I have done, you will never have to experience even one more day of feeling powerless and hopeless over your own obesity.

One of the most profound statements that Dr. Simeone's wrote that hit me hard and went right to my heart was: "The problems of obesity are perhaps not as dramatic as cancer, but they often cause lifelong suffering." This has definitely been true for me and describes what my life had been like.

CHAPTER 9

The Weight Loss Cure

So what is this miraculous plan that finally helped me to remove all the "abnormal fat deposits" from my body, increase my metabolism, and reach my goal weight?

I'm going to give a brief synopsis of this plan, so you my readers, will know the basics of this program and what you can expect.

However, since my book mostly involves my personal experiences and what I have done to achieve the beautiful, slim body that I now have, I want to refer you to check out and read Kevin Trudeau's book: "The Weight loss Cure'. There you will be able to read the entire regimen to follow, all the specifics of the plan, and decide for yourself if it's something that you want to do.

It is also very important to be aware that since "The Cure" comes from Dr. Simeone's "Weight Loss Cure protocol" which is detailed in his original manuscript; "Pounds and Inches: a New Approach to Obesity", you must also be sure to read this. After you read my book, if you are interested in following this plan for yourself, find this manuscript and read it in its entirety.

Dr. Simeone discusses in his manuscript, that while following the HCG treatment protocol, our bodies would lose all the "abnormal fat stores" and find a stable weight and at that point would not allow us to lose any more. He also wrote, that after HCG treatment, we should be able to eat well and find a stable maintenance weight, as long as we keep following the outlined regimen.

The protocol to follow consists of 4 separate Phases and each phase has a specific food plan with suggestions to follow.

PHASE 1 takes 30 days to complete. It involves using various cleanses to rid your body of toxins and stresses, cleansing your liver, colon and other organs, and to stimulate your lymphatic system. It is also supposed to help handle some of your nutritional deficiencies and correct hormonal imbalances in the thyroid and pancreas.

Kevin's book stated that doing Phase 1 would have tremendous long-term benefits and for me that has been proven true.

PHASE 2 is designed to stimulate the hypothalamus to release the secure fat deposits in one's problem areas at an accelerated rate. The time frame is between 3-6 weeks. By the completion of this phase, you are supposed to notice a remarkable reshaping of your body. My reshaping was absolutely amazing and I also found that my energy level was higher and my hunger and appetite lower.

PHASE 3 lasts 3 weeks and is designed to reset the Hypothalamus and body weight set point. It is supposed to keep the weight off permanently. Kevin's book says that this phase guarantees that your body is corrected from the abnormal condition which caused the obesity in the first place.

PHASE 4 is for the rest of your life. It includes suggested dos and don'ts to keep your hypothalamus healthy and stable. Following this phase should keep you from returning to your previous overweight and obese condition.

PHASE 1

PHASE 1 Follows Pages 76-92 of Kevin Trudeau's Book, "The Weight Loss Cure"

What does someone think when starting this process? Specifically, what was I thinking?

When I started PHASE 1 in September 2007, there was a mixture of fear and excitement and hope. My fear and excitement translated into the simple question of "Is this really going to work?" My sense of hope was directly related to the statement in the book and manuscript; "There is a cure", but the doubt in my mind responded "Really?"

I had feelings of confusion, doubt and being completely overwhelmed when looking at all the items on the various lists. I wondered what parts were crucial and mandatory for me and which ones were just extraneous and helpful.

I decided to stay calm and keep it simple. I asked myself the simple question of: Where do I start?

The plan recommended that you do many things that are considered healthy for one's body and to heal you from within. Some of the main one's for me were:

- Do not use any man made sugar or artificial sweeteners, (only the natural sweetener, Stevia), minimize using carbonated drinks and ice cold drinks, eat only organic foods and
- Do not use the microwave.

There is a list of my suggested do's and don'ts in this book and a full list in Kevin's book.

As I considered this, I knew that I was already completely off of sugar, flour, caffeine and regular sodas for the last nine years with my FA Program. So, I started with giving up Sweet n' Low and decaf coffee and then purchased and installed a water filter on the kitchen faucet and the master bathroom shower. I re-read Kevin's book and Dr. Simeone's manuscript again, underlining whatever seemed important, and took notes like I was back in graduate school. Then I started the suggested supplements, and bought as many of the Organic foods I could find. I planned my meals and tried really hard to eat dinner by 7pm. It was interesting, but for me, one of the most difficult changes that I struggled with was stopping my use of our microwave.

It seemed that the next thing for me to do was to locate and buy a Rebounder, which I did. A Rebounder is a mini-trampoline that is small enough to fit in most rooms and allows you to exercise by jumping up and down. The book said that this would help move my body and drain my lymphatic system to keep things flowing and help maintain my health. I started using the rebounder once a day at first and then I increased it to two times a day, first thing in the morning and at night before dinner. Once I started this exercise regimen, I next asked around for some local references and got a referral, and added the suggested colonics.

One of the suggestions was to use all Organic foods and spices and "coral calcium sachets". I went to the health food store and found most of the spices and foods I needed to start Phase 2, but I could not find Kevin's suggested "coral calcium sachets". Although I was told I could find it at a health food store, I could not. At first, the clerk said she had not heard of it and was sure they did not carry it. Then she searched her entire store and found one solo bottle of coral calcium capsules in an order that was sent to her by error and she could not sell it, so she gave it to me. This seems to be one of the many mysteries of how life works for me. It seems that when I believe in something wholeheartedly, am on the right path for me, and am committed towards my goal, "The Universe" seems to give me what I truly need.

Right from the start of following the "Weight Loss Cure" program, using the suggested cleanses and following Phase 1, the pre-HCG Phase, I started noticing positive changes in my body just as I had read in the book. To my surprise after about 2 weeks following this plan, I was reminded of my only experience with a diet that ever truly worked for me as written.

Back in 1996, I took the medications, Fen-Phen in addition to a weight loss diet plan. After about five months of eating about 800 calories a day and taking the pills, I reached a very slim weight of 112-115 pounds. I looked shapelier than I had ever been in all my life. I felt happier and more energetic than ever before and my bouts of depression ended. I did notice, though, that the drugs made me feel "spacey and high" a lot of the time. I ignored the side effects, because I wanted to be thin so very much. However, as much as I loved being slim, the obsessions and hunger did come back as soon as I stopped taking the pills and I added back the flour products. Then, my weight began to come back on quicker than ever. I began eating a lot of fast food; including my favorites: pizza and ice cream and all kinds of sugar and flour products. Within days, my addiction came back full force.

My history of dieting had shown me that I was never able to maintain any healthy weight for long. Even when I came to FA and lost a lot of my excess weight, I eventually began gaining weight again. The same was true for me after following Fen-Phen.

When I was following PHASE 1 and reading Kevin's book over and over, I found myself mulling over many of the things he wrote in addition to the actual diet plan. I was open to learning and found many of the things he said thought provoking. One concern he talked a lot about was how he viewed the diet and food and pharmaceutical industries in our country. What he referred to in his book made me wonder whether the real reason Fen-Phen was taken off the market was just a politically motivated, lobbying ploy.

There were news stories at the time about the drugs causing heart problems in people, but I have to wonder what the real truth was. There are a lot of medications circulating out there that cause many side effects, including heart problems and the FDA has not taken them off the market, yet. Could Fen-Phen have been one answer to the obesity issue that put fear into "the Corporate and Pharmaceutical companies that run our country", and capitalize on us "fat people"? I imagine that this could be a wonderful research project or master's thesis for some industrious person out there.

I considered what Kevin wrote seriously because one of my Endocrine specialists, who is very well known and well respected, had told me that Fen-Phen was extremely effective for most of his patients, and he believed the drugs were safer than they were said to be. This endocrinologist, a brilliant man who specializes in treating medically difficult patients with thyroid problems, shared with me his personal belief that the FDA "jumped the gun", and took away "One of the most effective weight loss treatments I have ever seen in my 30 plus years of practice". He said he felt the FDA had exaggerated the number of patients being harmed by the drugs. He told me that he was very suspicious of the real motives behind taking it off the market. Perhaps it was a "political move", just like many of the possibilities that Kevin brought up in his book. However, since it is not my intention in this book to get into any political arguments about the diet industry, I will just leave you with those questions to ponder yourselves.

After about three weeks following Phase 1, I was doing as much as I could do: drinking the recommended teas, going for colonics, using the cleanses, walking four times per week, daily use of the rebounder, no microwave usage, no Advil or over the counter medications, eating organic foods where possible, and no artificial sweeteners with only the occasional use of Stevia. I actually began to feel better. I had less gas, less bloating, less constipation and was generally speaking, feeling happier overall. I was really surprised by just how much the colonics were improving my bowels.

I did have a specific concern, though, just as some of you may have when you read his book. The book mentioned that a menstruating woman could not be menstruating during certain times of the starting process. I was worried that I might need to hold off on starting Phase 2 until after my menses was over. However, I decided to just have faith and trust that it would all work out in my best interests and to jump in and stop fussing and worrying. When I got my period 4 days prior to the start of my HCG injections, my worry was over and I felt very fortunate and grateful. I could then continue on with the plan and start the Phase 2 injections.

Although I was all prepared to start the next phase, my anxiety and fear crept back in and I needed to take some time to re-read "The Weight loss Cure" book and speak to the medical staff at HCG medical for information and encouragement. Re-reading Kevin's book and the testimonials I heard from the HCG medical staff was the final incentive it took to give me the hope to keep moving forward and try a diet regimen one more time.

Here is a brief Timeline on the start of my process. It all began after I read "The Weight Loss Cure."

> ➢ **01 August**

>> I read Kevin Trudeau's book, titled "The Weight Loss Cure." The first suggestion I followed was to give up decaf and sweet and low. I had already stopped using caffeine, and eating any sugar and flour products.

>> I did not eat any fried foods, had never smoked and stopped taking prescription medications, or over the counter, (OTC) medicines.

>> **(Note: I was already abstinent in FA for 9 years on an estimated 1100 calorie food plan.)**

> ➢ **30 August**

>> I went for my 1st colonic treatment.

> ➢ **30 August**

>> I went for my blood tests in order to be evaluated by HCG Medical and for the 1st time in four years, when my weight started increasing, I felt real hope.

> ➢ **02 September**

>> I started taking the suggested detoxes and supplements and using no butter spray.

While on vacation, Labor Day week, I ate according to my FA food plan and included the suggested supplements and teas and made my upcoming plan. I planned how I could continue to take the supplements for the full month and shop for organic foods when I got home. I planned how I could follow the HCG Diet for the estimated 40 to 45 days.

When I returned from my vacation, I read Trudeau's 1st book, "Health Cures" for additional insight and information.

➤ 24 September

I purchased and carried the "E-sports" pendant, which was supposed to give me more energy.

➤ 29 September

I installed a purifying shower filter.

More specifically, here is a list of my process and what I did when following Kevin's book:

1. I had already stopped eating all flour and sugar products and eating large quantities of food for 9 years.

2. I already drank only filtered water, and after reading Kevin's book, I also began using it for making tea, cooking oatmeal, and for everything else.

3. I had given up drinking any decaf coffee, all additives and dietary sweeteners, including sweet and low, aspartame in lozenges, gum and salad dressings, stopped using butter spray, and had switched to using sea salt.

4. I bought and used the suggested cleanses and supplements, including special teas and vitamins.

5. I bought a rebounder and used it 1-2 times a day.

6. I went for Colonics regularly.

7. I began looking for organic foods, but found this was one of the hardest parts of the regimen for me to follow. Organic foods were extremely costly and many were difficult to find.

8. I stopped using the microwave and tried to learn how to cook differently. I used a steamer, a pressure cooker, cooked on the stove in a saucepan, began using a teapot again and bought a George Forman grill.

9. I bought organic spices and eventually switched to using them regularly.

10. I ordered a shower water filter and an E-Sports pendant.

11. I bought a toaster oven, which I must admit; I only used occasionally during the diet and abandoned it afterwards.

12. I picked up my HCG prescription at CVS as soon as it came in. [Although, when I had to do a 2nd round of Phase 2 with the HCG, the company had changed their protocol and was dispensing it through their compounding pharmacy via the mail.]

13. I tried to eat my dinner by 6pm -6:30pm as was suggested, although I could not seem to follow this regimen every day. Due to my work schedule, I seemed to be sitting down for dinner around 7 pm many nights.

14. When the weather was nice, I walked 3-4 times a week, but when it was too cold out, I did not.

15. Per the protocol's instruction, I had completed taking all the suggested cleanses during Phase 1 and into the start of Phase 2, including: Candida Cleanse, Heavy Metal cleanse, Muscle Detox and the Colon cleanse. I had also completed the Fibermax and the Digest Max and tried the suggested whole food supplement. This was completed 1 week prior to starting my HCG injections

You will become very familiar with these cleanses after you read the book and start your own process.

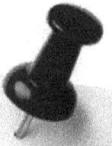

PHASE 2 is designed to stimulate the hypothalamus to release the secure fat deposits in one's problem areas at an accelerated rate. The time frame is between 3-6 weeks.

PHASE 2

PHASE 2 Follows Pages 92-98 of Kevin Trudeau's Book, "The Weight Loss Cure"

What I will now share with you is from the weight loss protocol in the original manuscript titled; "Pounds and Inches: A new approach to Obesity", by Dr. A. T. W. Simeons, MD, and book, titled, "The Weight Loss Cure" by Kevin Trudeau.

PHASE 2 is designed to stimulate the hypothalamus to release the secure fat deposits in one's problem areas at an accelerated rate. The time frame is between 3-6 weeks. By the completion of this phase, you are supposed to notice a remarkable reshaping of your body. In addition to my body being reshaped, I also found that my energy level was higher and my hunger and appetite lower.

This is the phase where you inject yourself with HCG, (Human Chorionic Gonadatrophin), first thing in the morning. It lasts from 21 days to a maximum of 45 days and you MUST do this phase under the supervision of a licensed health care practitioner following very specific guidelines, which are well outlined in Kevin Trudeau's book, "The Weight Loss Cure."

(Author's Note- Now in 2014, there is also the availability to get HCG drops instead of injections that seems to also be very effective for weight loss.)

PHASE 2 goes on for about 6 weeks and it's written that during this time you should lose approximately 1 pound per day.

The weight loss comes from your problem area secure fat deposits and your body becomes reshaped. My personal experience was that although it says one should lose one pound per day, I did not lose as much as the book stated. However, I lost a good amount of my excess weight, much more than any other diet I had ever followed, except Fen-Phen, and much of it was from my chunky, cellulite thighs and dimpled, fat derriere.

If you need to lose more weight after you complete the 45 days, you are told to take 6 weeks off, eating normally with the exception of no sugar or flour. It is also suggested that you be sure to eat enough protein so as not to develop a protein deficiency.

After this 6 week intermission, you can then resume another round of the phase 2 protocol for another 6 weeks. Now, if after this 2nd PHASE 2 process, if you still need to lose additional weight, then you must take off 8 weeks before starting a third round of the PHASE 2 protocol.

Now once you have completed one or more 6 week, (45 day) rounds of PHASE 2, and have lost all your excess weight while reshaping your body to your satisfaction, then you can proceed to PHASE 3.

Let me mention here that since my "malfunctioning" metabolism seemed to lose weight at about one-half the rate of other people, I ended up needing to follow Dr. Simeone's Phase 2 protocol twice; that's two times with HCG, in order to get all my excess weight off. However, ultimately all the weight did come off.

Personal Experiences from My Journal for Phase 2

These experiences below are from the first time that I followed PHASE 2 and took the HCG injections as advised in the "Weight Loss Cure" Program. I think it is important for me to relate my first few days' experiences with my readers, so that you will know what you can expect, know that it can be done and reassure you that it goes by quickly.

Monday, September 24th

Today was my first HCG injection day. In order to not make any mistakes, I read the instructions again, mixed up the HCG solution, and gave myself my 1st shot in the stomach. I was really afraid that it would hurt, but to my surprise, it did not. I had a lot of excess fat and I placed the needle in my skin, as directed, while I pinched the fat between my fingers. Now with that part done, I was able to relax a bit and know that I would be able to continue injecting myself daily. I spent a good part of that day thinking about following the instructions to eat excess food on my 1st "splurge day", as the book called it. This was a very difficult day for me. I had spent the last 9 years, working my FA program for food addiction, where I weighed and measured ALL my food before eating anything and that kept my obsession with food at bay. I had felt "neutral" about food for quite a while. For years, I had eaten either three weighed and measured meals each day or five smaller weighed and measured meals with nothing in between. Although, I did need to eat low calorie and low fat foods, including low fat proteins, in order to maintain my weight loss. I ate very few high calorie fruits or proteins, rarely ate cheese and never ate any dried fruits or any sugar or flour products.

It felt extremely uncomfortable for me. I was diligently following Phase 2 of the HCG plan, and being advised to eat "fattening, high calorie foods all day long". I understood the purpose was for my body to have enough energy source available when I started the 500 calorie food plan, and until the HCG started working in my system. I thought carefully about how to do what I was told and still maintain my Abstinence in FA.

(Note: Abstinence in FA is defined a weighed and measured meals with nothing in between, and no sugar or flour or any individual binge foods.) After much reflection and consultation with others, I chose to eat cheese, bananas and dates as my snacks during the day and I went out for a full meal at lunch. I had been eating such a limited and low calorie food plan for such a long time that following this regimen felt like I was eating just to eat. I noticed immediately that I rarely felt hungry as I had the last 3 weeks while following Phase 1.

All I wanted at the time was to get through the two "splurge" days and begin the HCG diet plan. I had to pray that those 2 days would give my body enough calories, so that I would not be hungry when I started the 500 calorie diet. I also stopped taking my thyroid medication per my interpretation of the protocol in the book. However, it's important to note here that later on that month, when I checked in with an HCG representative, I was told to resume my thyroid medication. It seems that I had misinterpreted their suggestion about taking prescription medications.

This misunderstanding, reminds me to warn the reader to be sure to ask all your questions to the medical provider guiding you while on this diet. There are no foolish questions and you must keep yourself healthy and safe at all times. I urge you to always be your own health care advocate, even if you feel you're being pushy and demanding.

It was at this time that I took the E-Pendant that I had bought, and began carrying it around in my pocket. The E-pendant is supposed to have some ability to change the magnetic force and energy surrounding the person wearing it. Supposedly, it could help increase my metabolism and possibly also my weight loss. Truthfully, I had a lot of doubts about whether this was valid or could work, but like I stated earlier, I was going to follow the complete protocol as closely as I could. To this day I still have questions and doubts about whether it helped me or not, but all my abnormal fat deposits came off and have stayed off, so I would have to say it was worth doing it for my peace of mind.

The decision I had made was to follow the plan with the same honesty, determination, and commitment that I had given to my FA program for the last 9 yrs.

Tuesday, September 25th

On the second "splurge' day, I weighed in at 144 pounds, took my supplements, gave myself a shot and then jumped for 10 minutes on my rebounder.

My food plan was a follows: I ate cheese with bananas for breakfast and for my snack, cheese, dates and oatmeal for lunch, and for dinner I had potatoes, cheese and chicken with blue cheese dressing. I felt quite full and almost stuffed most of the day. This was certainly a lot more food than I had been eating. I got through the day by reminding myself that the purpose was so I would NOT be hungry for the first week. I must say I did not like the feeling of being "stuffed". It reminded me of how I used to feel prior to following my FA program. Even though I had decided when I started PHASE 2, that I would treat it like a medical treatment, I knew I would be relieved when the next day came and I could start the 500 calorie diet. I thought that when I ate less food the next day, I could get my mind off thinking about how much I needed to be eating, get the excess weight off and begin to feel comfortable in my body again.

Not surprising to me, at 9:30 pm that night, I felt slightly nauseous from having eaten so much food throughout the day. I was even afraid that I would gain some weight when I weighed myself the next morning. The protocol suggests that we weigh ourselves each morning at the same time, in order to determine your status. This whole process was quite interesting to me. I never liked getting on a scale for fear of what weight I would be, but this process allowed me to develop neutrality around the entire issue and most days I would see a weight loss. I was so ready to start. Like I mentioned earlier, I had already begun feeling so much happier and healthier before these 2 splurge days. It was pretty amazing to me that I had felt more energetic, emotionally calmer, and had lost some weight, after one month of just taking the suggested cleanses.

Wednesday, September 26th

On the third day I weighed 145 and ½ lbs. and started the 500 calorie HCG diet plan. It felt wonderful to finally start the diet that I had read about for so long. I had been such a good dieter for so many years and I was ready. I bet many of my readers can identify with me that once we make up our minds to start a diet, we just want to jump in and do it.

The night prior, I experienced one of the worst nights that I had gone thru in a long time. I went to bed feeling some nausea and a little ill and afraid that I had reignited my food addiction. I sweated all night, had trouble falling asleep, and was restless the entire night. When I woke up, I felt what I would describe as "drugged" from too much food, and when I weighed myself, I had gained 1 and ½ lbs. Since I had expected the weight gain, I was not particularly surprised, but I hoped that it meant that I would be less hungry the next few days while the HCG kicked in.

I injected the HCG and drank a lot of purified water and suggested teas. I felt hungry until I got to work and actually felt much better than the day before when I was force feeding myself. I ate my organic apple at 11AM, and felt refreshed and then ate my lunch at 1pm and felt even better. During the day, I drank my teas, and ate my second apple when I was finishing up at work around 6:15pm. It was then that I realized that I was getting hungry. I went home and ate my dinner at 7:45pm. Then I rebounded again for 10 minutes and went to bed feeling slightly dizzy from jumping and a bit hungry. I must say, that I felt very positive and hopeful and so much better than the day before.

Thursday, September 27th

I had another difficult night and woke up at 4:15am and couldn't really go back to sleep. I did meditation and read a book and finally got up at 5am. I was feeling tired and somewhat "fuzzy" and sort of dizzy since 4:15am. I thought, "Let me just get through the day and hopefully get a good night's sleep tomorrow."

First thing I did when I finally got up on day 4 was to give myself my HCG injection. I noticed how much easier this was for me, and it made me appreciate just how many diabetics in the world have to do this every day. I also thought about how I have heard that some heroin addicts actually enjoyed shooting up and I wondered just what made someone get addicted to this process. I knew for sure that I definitely wasn't one of them. It is so interesting how our minds work and the thoughts that come into them. Of course, it could also be the result of too little sleep and my mind kind of wandering.

This fourth day, I was actually feeling excited to get on the scale, something I had been distressing over for almost two years, since I had reached 145 lbs. It was so nice to think of the scale with a positive vibe for a change. I also noticed that my intestines felt a little blocked and I was constipated and realized it was a direct consequence of what I had eaten the past two splurge days. I remembered the expression: "You are what you eat", and had to laugh. I went for a colonic and a massage. Both seemed to help a lot and made me feel better. I did notice, though, that all day I felt pretty hungry.

Friday, September 28th

I had a much better night's sleep and right from the start, I started feeling more energy. The discipline of weighing myself regularly for the first time in years increased my feelings of strength and hope. It was a real shock to me and yet a pure thrill, when I noticed that I was actually shedding some excess weight. For the first time in 2 years, I saw weight come off my body. It was amazing to me, that I was actually getting some weight loss. It all began with my taking the suggested cleanses and having regular colonics, and continued now that I was following phase 2. This was something I never would have believed and it amazed me. The hope and excitement I felt, brought tears of joy to my eyes. I found myself so emotional, that I cried every time I talked to my husband about it.

Saturday, September 29th

Today, I read the HCG injection directions for the 10th or 15th time and realized that I was still nervous and anxious about doing it correctly. I knew I was making too much out of it all, but I wanted the shots to work for me. As a dentist I inject my patients every day at work, but injecting myself while desperately wanting the treatment to work, built up a lot of anxiety for me.

For the rest of Phase 2, I carried on pretty much the same every day with all the emotional ups and downs expected. Having renewed hope and a disciplined plan to follow, I was living each day the best I could. Looking back now, I can see that I carried on like a trooper with excitement and anticipation of watching the pounds melt off my body and leaving me thinner and happier.

PHASE 2-THE SECOND TIME AROUND

When I realized I hadn't lost all the weight I needed to lose, I did what was outlined in Kevin's book, page 96. I took 6 weeks off and resumed my normal FA food plan, which followed the protocol of No sugar or flour, ordered another prescription of HCG, and followed Phase 1 again for another 6 weeks.

This second time went just like it had the first time, but I was much more aware of what to do and what to expect. I was worried that the injections would be painful this time around since my stomach was smaller and I had lost much of my excess fat. I was very relieved, when the injections felt no different than they did the first time around. However, It did seem like I was hungrier this second time and that I was more anxious to be done and get my excess fat off. I think that was very normal for anyone following any kind of "diet' and shows how impatient one can get and how we always want to move on to the next thing in life instead of "enjoying the journey". This could lead into a very interesting philosophical discussion, but I know that's not why you're reading this book, so I will move on.

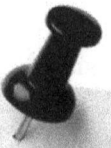

PHASE 3 goes on for 21 days, (three weeks), and although it is relatively simple, it also has a very specific protocol to follow.

PHASE 3

PHASE 3 Follows Pages 99-102 of Kevin Trudeau's Book, "The Weight Loss Cure"

PHASE 3 is a very important phase that is designed to reset the Hypothalamus and the body weight set point. It is supposed to keep the weight off permanently. Kevin's book says that this phase guarantees that your body is corrected from the abnormal condition which caused the obesity in the first place.

This is the phase where your body's metabolism gets reset to a high normal state, eliminates future intense and constant hunger, and prevents the abnormal future storing of fat in those secure problem area fat reserves in your body.

This phase goes on for 21 days, (three weeks), and although it is relatively simple, it also has a very specific protocol to follow.

You must weigh yourself every morning without fail! It takes about 3 weeks after completing Phase 2 before your weight will stabilize. If your weight stays within 2 pounds of the final Post-Injection day weight, you are in fine shape.

However, as soon as the scale goes beyond the 2 pounds, you must follow a very specifically outlined protocol to get those 2 pounds off. I lovingly call this the "Weight Loss Cure"- *Diet Steak Day* protocol. Kevin's book does an excellent job of giving specifics of this diet steak day as well as helpful hints and behavior changes to make Phase 3 work effectively and help you be successful.

Kevin says in his book that: "When you successfully complete the 21 days of Phase 3, you are ready to begin your new life as a normal, thin, energetic, happy, healthy person who is no longer a slave to hunger, food cravings and food."

My personal experience with Phase 3 was one of trial and error. I did the best I could to follow as much of the written suggestions from Kevin's book. However, I must be honest with you and say that some of the suggestions were almost impossible for me to follow exactly. Those that I had total control over, I did fairly well with. Those that involved other people, places or had some financial restraints, I did not follow completely.

I controlled my food intake very well and had absolutely No sugar or flour or starch, (as listed in his book), no artificial sweeteners, no fast foods at restaurants, no trans fats, no nitrates, no ice cold drinks and I limited my nonprescription and prescription medicines. I was unable to limit my total exposure to air conditioning and fluorescent lights due to my work environment and my outside activities where they involved other people's choices.

What else did I do? Let me list those suggestions that I followed and found very helpful:

- I drank about one gallon of pure spring water or purified water every day without the coral calcium sachets recommended, that no one at my local health food stores or at the online links could locate.

- I walked between 30 minutes to 1 hour on most Fridays, Saturdays and Sundays, and during the week when I had time and weather permitted.

- I tried to eat one apple every day, sometimes organic and other times not. I ate one grapefruit 2 to 3 times a week.

- I had raw organic cider vinegar on most days, but never ate any raw organic coconut.
- I drank Elotin tea every day and drank lots of organic, decaffeinated teas and used Stevia when sweetener was needed.
- I used a Three Lac substitute from the health food store. I also slept an average of seven hours a night. However, since I have a personal issue with insomnia, I tended to get up 3 to 4 times a night.
- I took Probiotics and Vitamin E every morning.
- I gave up ALL artificial sweeteners, stopped drinking decaf coffee, and used no ice at all.
- I used my rebounder for 10-15 minutes every morning and usually also at night.
- I went for a Colonic regularly and whenever I felt the need, I wore my E-pendant for energy and balance every day, I added cinnamon occasionally to my foods and had a salad at lunch and dinner on most days.
- I bought organic foods when possible, used sea salt and organic spices and never ate anything with MSG.
- I did my best to avoid creams, lotions or moisturizers and anything with the ingredients sodium laurel sulfate or propylene glycol, but sometimes it was unavoidable. We had already installed and used the home water filter and a shower filter, as mentioned earlier.
- I tried to use a toaster oven and George Forman grill, but ended up going back to using our microwaves after I completed PHASE 3 and thru most of Phase 4.
- I ate six small weighed and measured meals every day.

- I usually ate dinner around 7PM and went to bed between 9-10 PM. (I would try to eat at 5:30-6:00 PM, but my work schedule had me getting home at 6:30 many nights.)

I weighed myself every morning without exception and if I gained more than 2 pounds, I followed the exact protocol of the "diet steak and apple day" that's listed on pages 101-102 from "The Weight Loss Cure".

Now, to make sure you keep your newly corrected condition permanently and don't damage your Hypothalamus again, you must go immediately on to PHASE 4.

Phase 4 is the program for you to follow for the rest of your life.

HINT: *If you feel scared off or overwhelmed by all that's suggested to do, here is my must do list of what to do or what not to do during the process.*

- <u>Do not use a microwave</u>
- <u>Walk every day for 1 hour if possible</u>
- Use a Rebounder for at least 5-10 minutes twice a day
- Do not ingest any sugar or flour products
- Do not use any diet or artificial sweeteners
- Do not have any ice or drink any cold drinks that can slow up your metabolism.

If you can at least do these things to start your process, and allow yourself some time to feel better and to begin to feel successful, then maybe you will start being able to add more suggested items in each day.

PHASE 4

PHASE 4 Follows Pages 105-112 of Kevin Trudeau's Book, "The Weight Loss Cure"

Just like the other 3 phases, I followed Phase 4 as written in the book. However, over time, I had to adjust many of the suggestions to fit my lifestyle. I bought organic when I could find what I needed and when the cost was not what I would call exorbitant.

I ate only fresh or frozen foods and ate nothing with preservatives, additives or of a fast food variety. I did cleanses as needed for the first year and continued to follow much of what I wrote in Phase 3.

I found that I was unable to maintain my HCG final weight and I actually gained about 5 pounds that I was unable to reduce even after following 3 steak days in a 7 day period. I am sure this would not be a recommended, healthy suggestion by anyone following this plan, but I was determined to try it out and find a way to lose the gained weight.

Since I could not get these five pounds off, I decided to accept this new weight as my body's new "ideal, set point" goal weight. I have been able to maintain this weight and live a contented life following my FA food guidelines as my basic structure and using the Phase 4 principles and suggestions. I absolutely love my slim body and thin figure. I want to say again that I am so very grateful for finding Kevin's book and my own willingness to follow Dr. Simeone's protocol. I hope you decide to try it and I wish you the same success that I have had.

My personal opinion of Phases 1-4 is that they offer and deliver the "Promises" written in Kevin's book and what I would define as: "Truly a Miracle".

My hunger has become normalized and is not intense and constant. I can eat an "average" portion and be satisfied and full. My food cravings are gone. My metabolism seems to have reached a stable level for my body size and activity level. I have not stored any new abnormal fat deposits that I am aware of. Cellulite is a thing of the past!! I no longer suffer from the food related depression, stress or food anxiety. I no longer feel like a slave to food or imprisoned in a fat, "ugly" body!!

CHAPTER 10

Cleanse Day: Diet Steak Day

As I have already mentioned, when you gain more than 2 pounds, "The Weight Loss Cure" book tells you to immediately follow a "steak day". This is really very simple, but it is not that easy. By the time 1 pm rolls around, you will probably be feeling hungry, a little bit edgy and wanting to eat something. The first time I did this, I was able to get thru my day, but it was extremely stressful and it affected my mood, energy output and productivity. However, it got a little easier, the more I did it. I love being in a thin body so much and I want to stay thin so desperately that it has been more than worth it for me. As a matter of fact, when I follow thru completely with these diet days, it actually makes me feel "cleaner" inside, almost like a "body cleansing".

Over time, I have been able to have less steak days and keep my body weight stable on my regular food plan. It's important for my readers to remember that I have ALWAYS had a metabolism that gains weight very oddly. You are much more likely to find your weight staying relatively stable and not needing to turn to a diet steak day very often.

One of the amazing aspects of this steak day is that even after eating a large portion of steak, with either 8oz of tomatoes or a large apple for dinner; I would wake up the following day, weigh myself and actually be right back on track. How my body can readjust itself like this still continues to baffle me and feels like a miracle. Speaking of miracles and I really cannot say this enough, the entire "Weight Loss Cure" Program seems like a miracle to me.

It is now over six years since I first followed "The Weight Loss Cure". I continue to maintain my weight by following the Phase 4 protocol alongside my FA food plan. I have found that I still need to do an occasional diet steak day. However, I have had to make a slight adjustment to the protocol in order to be able to function well and get through the day effectively.

I used to drink lots of diet soda or chew sugarless gum during the day, but I began overdoing it and realized it was not helping my hunger very much. So now I allow myself one or two apples at lunch to tide me over till dinner.

This has caused me NOT to lose 2 full pounds, but it has made my following Phase 4 much more manageable while still maintaining my weight. I think once you reach PHASE 4 and follow it for a while, you will need to reassess your own personal status and how your body responds and decide what YOU can honestly follow for the rest of your life.

CHAPTER 11

COLONICS

This is a necessary topic for the complete "Weight Loss Cure" plan to work and give you the results promised. For those of you, who have never had a colonic, let me share my experience with you and include all the nitty, gritty details.

When Kevin's book suggested colonics, I thought: "You've got to be kidding!" I once had a colonoscopy and I was not planning on having anyone "stick another tube in my rear end" any time soon. However, I was going to stay open-minded. I had made the commitment to follow his book 100% and to do so to the best of my ability.

I had read about colonics over the years and thought they were mainly for unhealthy people that had gastrointestinal issues and were "filled with shit" and unable to have any bowel movements. I had assumed they were recommended for medical problems like irritable bowel syndrome or spastic colon disease.

So, I researched it some more, located a local colonics therapist and realized that I actually had many of the symptoms that warranted my undergoing colonics treatments. I never wanted to spend much time thinking about my bowels, but after consulting with Pam, the colonic therapist, I began to acknowledge that I had actually spent a lifetime being somewhat embarrassed and limited by my bouts of constipation and chronic gas. This included when I used to diet and even after I had joined

FA, where I ate a large salad and cooked vegetables for lunch and dinner every day.

Pam told me that constipation and bowel issues affect more people than I had ever imagined. Once again, I was Not alone nor unique. You, too, may not be! Until she told me this information, I had never gone to a pharmacy or department store just to check out the section with all the many antacids and bowel/intestinal gas regulators. When I went to the store to check it out as she had suggested, I was absolutely amazed how many rows upon rows of products there were.

Anyway, I must warn you, the 1st colonic can be quite the experience. When I went for my first appointment, I was told to lie on a cotton sheet on a table, and Pam then inserted a plastic tube with Vaseline on it just where you'd expect and covered me with a large towel. Yes, I did feel extremely vulnerable and embarrassed. Pam did make me feel as comfortable as she could and acted like a true medical professional. I liken the feeling I had during the process to women's physical PMS symptoms or having menstrual cramps. It was not painful to me as I had anticipated, just odd and uncomfortable. It was actually very humbling.

The remarkable thing was that it really helped. As I lay there on her table, trying not to be uptight and meditating on "letting go", I began to feel "less stuck" and soon noticed how much flatter my stomach became. The entire process intrigued me and I wondered what I'd feel like after the session was completed.

The truth is that immediately afterward, and for the remainder of the day my stomach was slightly uncomfortable, I felt somewhat "bloated" and I had to eat a light diet. However the following day and for some time after, my body felt lighter, my stomach was flatter and I had less gas, less cramping and much less discomfort from constipation.

I was fortunate to have been referred to a fantastic and skilled colonics therapist who is a kind and understanding woman with a wealth of information that she was willing to share.

As I mentioned earlier, I learned that a multitude of people in our society have bowel issues that probably relate to the poor diet and poor eating habits we have as a society in the US, in addition to most people's busy and stressful lives. It seems many of us hold our stress inside and if you tend to have a susceptible nervous system, you may be prone to bowel problems like constipation, "bloating" or gas.

Interestingly enough, as I continued to have additional colonics sessions, I began to remember the many times in my past that constipation had plagued me. I somehow had forgotten them or blocked them out from denial due to shame. I even began to wonder if perhaps, at one time in my past, I had developed a spastic colon.

One strong suggestion for those of you just starting your search for a colonic therapist; be sure to check them out thoroughly. Call them and meet with them first for a consult. Ask a lot of questions!! Ask them how long they have done it, what type of disposables and sterilization they use, what techniques they plan for you, how much time it will take and what their fees are. I would suggest that you find one that uses purified water (since it will be entering into YOUR body), uses ONLY disposables and has a lot of experience and knowledge. Most importantly, be sure that you choose a therapist that you feel comfortable and safe with and that their techniques are sound.

When all is said and done, when you try colonics, I believe you will agree with me and say that you feel healthier, lighter and glad that you added colonics to your health regime.

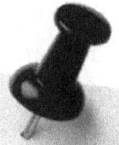

During Phase 1 and 2, I had very little trouble with my bowels, probably because there was so little food going in, so of course not much coming out. But as I entered Phases Three and Four, the same old problem returned.

CHAPTER 12

Constipation

Now here is a fun topic that must be addressed. Most diets do not discuss what could happen to one's digestive processes while changing your diet and following their program. However, anyone that has gone on any type of diet knows that there are consequences when they make dietary changes. I have found that for me, I always need to address the issue of constipation at some point during the diet.

It seems that whenever I change what I put into my body, there are changes to the balance of how my body's many systems function. Occasionally some foods do not agree with me and I get gas or indigestion. I can get an acid stomach, feel bloated and uncomfortable, or I can have what could be classified as being "sensitive or allergic". Each of us will learn by our own process of trial and error just what specific foods, drinks, or spices cause these changes within us. For me bananas and cheese and rice will definitely harden up my stool, while grapes, cantaloupe, applesauce and decaf coffee will loosen up my bowels rather quickly.

One of the many things I love about the "Weight Loss Cure" plan is that it is written very clearly and with 4 specific phases describing the entire "have to do's" and the good suggestions that are healthy but not mandatory. I love definitive directions. When I become completely ready and willing to follow a suggested plan, I follow it exactly as it is written. Some may call it my perfectionist personality, but when I follow a plan that has been touted as proven to work and I follow it to the letter, I expect it to work for me. So many other programs, especially popular diets and "health regimes for weight loss" never even came close to working like the literature boasted about.

However, the "Weight Loss Cure" meets the mark. It works.

Well now, let us get back to constipation. I can now honestly admit that I have always had a very difficult time with my bowels and felt plagued by constipation. At times it has been either embarrassing or has caused me to limit my life and my activities.

During Phase 1 and 2, I had very little trouble with my bowels, probably because there was so little food going in, so of course not much coming out. But as I entered Phases Three and Four, the same old problem returned. I found I had to depend on my colonics appointments like a "medicine" that I would need to take regularly for my bowels to function well. I even began to worry that I would need to plan my life to have colonics weekly in order to maintain my weight and my health. I knew that it was worth considering, but I was determined to find a less costly solution and hopefully one I could have more control over.

Well, after being willing to share this very intimate and humiliating topic with a few close friends I found the most wonderful solution. It gave me back a healthy, fully functioning bowel and put me back in control. It is called H2Go by Lane Labs. It is a bottle of "pills" with directions to start by taking six, then five, then four until you learn exactly what amount your own body needs to digest the foods you eat. It is <u>NOT</u> a drug! It is only Active Magnesium. It metabolizes and is absorbed within your colon and allows water to enter the colon system and loosen up the bowels, thereby eliminating your wastes in a gentler manner.

However, I must caution you. You can overdo it and find out you are now "stuck" with the problem of diarrhea and will need to be close to a bathroom. I decided to follow my rule of thumb, go slowly and each night consider what I ate that day and determine how many tablets to take before retiring for the night. You will figure it out very quickly. For me it released me from the burden of constipation and gave my life more freedom.

It worked in the beginning and it continues to do what it is supposed to do many years later. So, if you find you are burdened by constipation, order a bottle and try it, you will be glad you did!

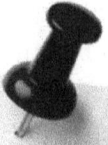

It never ceases to amaze me that when I allow myself to be open-minded and willing to try something new, I very often end up liking it and wishing I had tried it sooner.

CHAPTER 13

Thoughts on Exercise and the Rebounder

To my way of thinking, there is a big difference between exercising for health and strength and exercising for weight loss. Not only do I hate exercise, but I am physically "sports challenged" and have little desire and limited energy for a lot of it. So when I read Kevin's suggestion that I should use a rebounder five to ten minutes a day in the morning and evening, I was not very excited about it, but I did think that it might be doable for me. It was recommended because using a rebounder helps drain our lymphatic system, allowing us to be healthier.

Since it was such a small requirement, I thought that I could probably do it and maybe even be successful at it and keep it up daily. I entertained the thought, that it might even be fun to jump and down to music and maybe it would help me reduce my stress while helping my health.

So I bought one, used it and found out that I actually liked it. As a matter of fact, the first rebounder I got was a low-cost one, since I was concerned it would be another gadget that I would buy and never use. Well, what a surprise when I got it, used it every day, and found out that I actually enjoyed it.

I played a CD with an upward beat, that I really liked and within a few months the springs failed and I had to get a new one. Then my husband did a little searching on the internet and bought a more expensive model for me. Today, I love using my rebounder. I find that I look forward, most days to getting on it for 10-15 minutes before I start my day. It seems to make me feel more virtuous and somewhat "athletic. I have even found that many days I use it as a "jumping meditation".

It never ceases to amaze me that when I allow myself to be open-minded and willing to try something new, I very often end up liking it and wishing I had tried it sooner. So my advice to you is to give the rebounder a try and see for yourself. Who knows, it might end up being something you add to your exercise ritual just for fun and stress relief.

CHAPTER 14

Testing My Limits, My Metabolism and My Hypothalamus

Learning how to eat to maintain my thin body has been challenging to say the least.

As far back as I can remember, I have had an unhealthy fear of food. I would constantly worry about what foods I could eat, what quantity would satisfy me and whether it should be a low calorie, "diet food" or not. I always chose diet dressings, since I thought that healthy oils had too many calories. As I already told you, when I followed my 12 Step suggested food plan, I lost a lot of weight over time, but could never take off the last twenty pounds. My weight got stuck between 140-145 pounds and would not budge. I tried eating less, (800 to 1000 calories per day), but I still stayed stuck at 140-145 pounds. When the food plan was increased to 1200 calories, in accordance to my nutritionist's advice, I gained weight. My nutritionist was baffled; because she told me my metabolic index indicated that I needed 1263 calories per day for my basic functions without any additional activity. My response to her was: "Why then was I still overweight?" She had absolutely no answer for me and I became frustrated and upset.

So, after following the "Weight Loss Cure" plan and finally losing all my excess weight, I was in a thin body and determined to stay that way no matter what. Kevin's book clearly stated that after I reached my final goal weight, I would be able "to eat whatever I wanted, as long as I stopped when I was full" and weighed myself daily. His book said that when my weight became two pounds over, then I should immediately follow his outlined "steak day", and the additional weight would come off.

It sounds so simple, doesn't it? I'm sure it would be for a "normal eater", but remember I have identified myself as a recovering food addict. I have limitations and restrictions that must be followed or I can get into some serious difficulties.

I knew from my experience of being a food addict that I would never really be able to eat "everything I wanted", and that I almost never felt totally "full", unless I had already overeaten. What I was hoping for was a way to eat regular, healthy, satisfying meals and maintain a slim body and clear mind. I was also convinced that my Hypothalamus had definitely corrected itself to some degree but that I still had a relatively sluggish metabolism, including my digestive and bowel systems.

When I first began my FA program over 15 years ago, I ate two large salads, two servings of cooked vegetables, 3 servings of protein, and 1-2 fruits a day. I have learned that eating the three full-sized meals like the majority of my FA Fellowship does will make me feel too stuffed, bloated, and unable to function well. After losing my abnormal fat deposits by way of the HCG plan, three full meals were definitely too much bulk for me. Besides not feeling good, it could cause me to gain almost two pounds within two to three days, no matter what the calories added up to. I also knew that I felt so much better when I ate five or six smaller meals throughout the day.

So, when I started Phase 4, I tried to follow the book's suggested food plan, but I noticed that on some weeks when I ate what was described as "normal", I could gain about 2 pounds in a week. My weight started off at 112-115 pounds, and after 5-6 days, my weight had crept up to 116-118 pounds. This had gone over the two pound limit, and I was supposed to immediately follow a diet steak day. I did what was suggested and the "diet steak day" miraculously worked, but the next time it happened, I thought I could compensate for it by cutting back my daily food plan. However, the next week, I still regained two pounds and I found myself feeling hungry during the day and waking up at night thinking a lot about food.

So then I tried the book's suggestion to eat some weighed out chicken before going to bed, or to eat my snack fruit at night when I felt particularly hungry and had eaten lightly all day. However, there seemed no definite consistency with my weight. Some weeks I would gain weight and other weeks my weight stayed stable. This led me to planning a "diet steak day" once a week. I justified it to myself by calling it a "cleanse" day". This was relatively easy in the beginning, but over time it got so much more difficult. In order to not get overly frustrated and anxious, I decided that I needed to be patient and give my metabolism time to re-adapt.

Eventually, after trying a lot of food plans, I was able to come up with one that gives me enough variety, keeps me well nourished, keeps away all food cravings and lets me stay thin at around 118-122 pounds. I believe that my hypothalamus has re-set itself at a new "Set Point" causing me to gain a few more pounds. For me to be content, I have accepted this slightly higher post-HCG weight and the reality of my body's wisdom. I have also accepted the fact that I still have to do an occasional diet steak day, in order to keep what I have. I am extremely grateful that so far, I have been willing to keep following this plan that allows me to maintain my slim, shapely body.

When I analyzed what had been causing me some of my problems early on in the process, I realized that I was getting into trouble when I would plan to eat very light during the day due to the fact that I felt so much better eating lighter and I had a hectic work schedule. Some days I would get caught up in my work and even though I was hungry around three or four in the afternoon, I would think I could skip my afternoon snack and wait until dinner. Then, if I had a class at night or a meeting to go to, I would come home at 7pm for dinner and I would be almost starving. Since I could only eat so much bulk at a single meal and still feel physically comfortable, I would eat only a small dinner meal thinking that I would have the rest as my evening snack. However, by the time I was ready to retire for bed, it seemed too late to eat a snack and I would talk myself out of it, deciding I did not need it.

Then as you might expect, I would wake up hungry a couple of hours after going to bed and I would think about having my snack. I could justify eating it by telling myself that I had skipped my snacks during the day, that it was my committed food, and that eating my snack would help me to go back to sleep. It was just so easy for me to justify that I had planned to eat this food earlier in the day, that I was hungry and tell myself that "I could always follow a "diet steak day", if I needed to. But when I did decide to eat my planned snack, I would feel very guilty and not want to let my sponsor or my husband know about it. This horrible guilt came from my past history of being a sleep eater which was a very difficult period in my life. I understood that when I started to feel all this guilt, it could lead me to other types of dishonesty with food and set off more of my addictive behaviors, which could ultimately lead me to overeat and break my commitment to Abstinence.

Many years before I followed the "Weight Loss Cure", I would wake up a lot at night due to the effects of Perimenopause, Menopause and the related insomnia problem, and needing to go to the bathroom a lot in the middle of the night. This led to my developing a habit of getting up at night, feeling hungry and either fighting off wanting to eat or giving in to my hunger. It became such a disturbing dilemma for me where I felt I was fighting a battle with myself every night. I did not want to repeat that way of living ever again.

I could also see that this type of thinking had the possibility to become an "addict's trap". Knowing my addictive past, I realized that this habit and my feeling of wanting to be secretive about my food, was not a healthy way for me to carry on. Gratefully, I realized this pretty quickly and knew I had to find a better way.

What I finally chose to do and still do now is to eat all my planned meals during my waking hours. When I wake up at night, I stay in my bedroom no matter how hungry I am. I also do not allow myself to buy any trigger food or "personal binge foods" that will set me up for any dysfunctional habit to take hold. So far this system has solved any late night eating dilemma before it could get out of hand.

I am pretty sure that a lot of my difficulties were specific to my lifelong issues with my metabolism and my food addiction. I hope that you will not experience these same challenges. I would expect that your process will be much easier and more in tune with what Dr. Simeone and Kevin's experiences have shown.

I have completely accepted that I will always need to be very careful with what I eat, and take in fewer calories than what the nutritionist, health/weight guidelines and all the metabolic formulas say I need. I can only hope that as more research comes forward and more proof comes to light, that new books and articles and guidelines will be written that give us more accurate information and that people in general, especially thin ones, stop assuming that all fat people are weak willed or lying about what they eat.

Speaking of this, I have been feeling very encouraged with new research that has been coming to light. This research has been confirming what so many of us have already known for many years; we just didn't have the proven facts from scientific studies to give us credibility. Research I have read that goes back to January 2012 showing that they have discovered many hormones that are associated with fat, weight gain and loss, and hunger. They have finally discovered many biochemical pathways in our bodies that control and ultimately determine our food cravings, our set point weight and ultimately how effective and efficient our metabolism will be for each of us individually.

The research is proving that once someone has gained and lost weight a few times or had the "yoyo" diet cycle, that their metabolism has actually been re-set and has truly changed causing them to lose weight slower, gain weight faster and need to either eat less food or have more active exercise in order to stay at a previous thinner body weight. For so many years, many heavy women and those of us previously fat women have said that we eat less and seem to gain more weight than the amount of calories we take in or that we eat less than our thin friends and they stay thin and we keep gaining weight. We have been looked at with disbelieving eyes, even from our physicians and nutritionists.

I wish there had been a book that had outlined a solution to help me along my journey. I have done my best to offer this type of book to you, but since each of us is slightly different, you will each need to experiment and find out what works best for you. My suggestion is that once you reach your goal weight, each of you should find your own personal food plan and "take what you need and leave the rest" from mine.

That is why I decided to write this book. I wanted to offer all my personal experiences and successes and failures, hoping that it would help someone else. Let me have done all the difficult and at times painful research for you. Believe me when I tell you that if you have been unable to lose weight or if those last 20-30 pounds just will not come off, you need to try the "Weight Loss Cure".

The bottom line is: you have nothing to lose except your abnormal fat deposits!

Believe in yourself and that you DESERVE to be healthy, thin and enjoy your life fully.

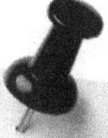

These were the times when I hadn't planned out my day well and made poor choices about my food; planning to eat less during the day usually because of my poor digestion.

CHAPTER 15

Just Say No! Combining My FA Structure with "The Weight Loss Cure" Program

Since no one I knew in FA had followed the "Weight Loss Cure" plan before me, I could find no sponsor as a mentor or guide. As I said previously, I saw myself as being a "maverick" going down new paths and needing to "find my own way." I knew that I had done this many times before in other areas of my life and that I had come through just fine. I had even flourished in some aspects of my life. It looked like once again the upward hill would be my personal journey. Although it was a very fearful and uncertain time for me I was very hopeful and wanted to believe that I was making a breakthrough.

Following Kevin's book gave me the way to lose my extra weight, but I still had to review his suggestions and determine what combinations would keep me thin for a lifetime. I was determined to keep the wonderful results that I had achieved, no matter what! I knew that my body and how it metabolized food was still different from many others in my FA program.

When I started Phase 4, I worked with my FA sponsor and ate her suggested "planned out, daily food plan" of 3 regular

FA meals, but I gained two pounds within the first week as I wrote earlier in this book. So then I tried a suggested plan of six smaller meals, but in a few weeks I once again gained a couple of pounds. It seemed like I could NOT follow the same food plan that others she knew followed and maintain a stable weight. So I used a suggestion from Kevin's book and ate five or six small meals, weighed daily and when I was over my basic weight by two pounds, I did the suggested diet steak day. I noticed however, that occasionally I felt bloated and uncomfortable. It seemed that at times my body had difficulty digesting and metabolizing and I would gain weight. So, I began my plan to follow a "diet steak day" about once a week.

This caused my food addiction mindset to creep back in and I began thinking about dieting and fasting. In order to combat this I had to stay very diligent about keeping my combined commitments to my Abstinence in FA and the "Weight Loss Cure" protocol. I never ate any sugar or flour and I weighed out my food portions, but there were times that I felt I had to "hang on for dear life". These were the times when I hadn't planned out my day well and made poor choices about my food; planning to eat less during the day usually because of my poor digestion. I realized pretty quickly that this was a poor decision, since it always set me up to fail. My sponsor quickly reminded me that I was unable to function well when I was hungry, and that I needed to be consistent and stay on my food plan.

Looking back, the early days were definitely challenging and I had to do a lot of "trial & error" food planning, in order to determine what would later become my "balanced, sane and contented" food plan. My willingness to be patient, work with my FA sponsors and trust in myself to try some different food plans, ultimately helped me to find a balanced food plan that fed my body nutritionally, kept the food cravings away and allowed me to live an enjoyable, contented, "thin" life.

As I said before, I am sure that my process was much more difficult than yours will be. However, I want to offer you hope that even with all the difficulties I experienced, the "Cure" still worked for me and I was able to obtain my goal of a thin body and maintain it years later.

Some might consider my disciplined way of eating as too restrictive or difficult, but for me it has become "the easier, softer way" for sure. I already told you that until recently, I had never gotten thin and stayed thin or had the chance to learn how to eat for this purpose. You have read that I have never had the type of metabolism that simply burned off calories and allowed me guilt free eating. I have always wanted more than my share and certainly more than my body could burn off in any given day. Even when I was on my disciplined FA food plan, I either gained a little over time or gained continuously and could never find a healthy, daily food plan that kept my weight stable. That is what contributed to my feeling guilty about food all the time and was certainly not a serene and joyful way to live.

What I know for sure is that for me to remain "Abstinent, Clean, and Sober" in FA, I must not put any sugar or flour into my body and I need to weigh out all my food portions to keep the quantities limited. It has been proven to me over and over, that in order for me to live a serene and content life, I must follow this rule no matter what. I have done this for over fifteen years and am convinced beyond a shadow of a doubt that this cannot change.

What I also know is that I need to "Say No" to any food that calls to me, makes me wish I could have more of it, or is reminiscent of any of my individual binge foods. It has been interesting for me to find that over time the foods that "call" to me change depending on where I am in my life, and what the status is of my emotional and spiritual recovery.

Even knowing this there have been a few days and especially some late nights, when I am tired and edgy and there seems to be a switch that goes off in my head and saying "NO" feels like the last thing I want to do. I can feel a strong urge to just want to react and eat or drink something as a coping mechanism to deal with life. In 12 Step circles we talk about "the Committee" in our heads, those voices that we hear that try to justify unhealthy behavior and suggest that we can "eat or drink just one, just this time". Those thoughts that tell us that after eating "just one" we won't want any more and all will be just fine. Saying "NO" may sound like a very simple suggestion, but for a food addict, it can be quite a challenge. My experience in my 12 Step programs has taught me that I cannot listen to these inner voices or act on any thoughts that suggest I do something that is not good for me and will absolutely sabotage all I have done.

So, I have trained myself to say "NO" to myself when my thoughts tell me to go off my program and take a chance that things will be different, "this time". I work very hard at not letting myself be tempted or giving in and I use all the tools my fellowship and 12 Step program have taught me. I have learned that each day I need to make a firm commitment to follow my FA recovery program and the Phase 4 protocol, get lots of outside help when needed and to always be willing to do what is necessary. I turn to my 12 Step fellowship regularly, use my "Power greater than myself" on a daily basis and keep a clear focus on my strong desire to stay in a thin body.

The bottom line for me as a food addict is that each one of us needs to figure out exactly what our individual bodies' need each day in order to keep us healthy, able to function well without any food obsession, and still stay thin. We MUST be entirely honest with ourselves and be willing to stop ourselves and say NO to picking up any food that calls to us or causes us to crave it and want more than we need. If you are not a Food Addict, you may find this quite easy. However, if you are a food addict and cannot stop yourself by saying "NO", then go ahead and check out your closest OA or FA Fellowship for support and help.

I know that it would have been so much easier for me if my FA sponsor could have given me a definite food plan, or if I could have found guidance in a book like I am now writing.

Unfortunately, no one had followed this path before me in FA and everyone I turned to for guidance told me they were clueless as to how to help me. Perhaps this book will offer such guidance for you.

My advice to my readers is to look at all your behaviors and be as honest as you possibly can. If you think you may be a Food Addict like me, talk to a trusted friend and share what you are doing. Then seek out a program to help you overcome it. My personal recommendation is to check out FA, Food Addicts in Recovery Anonymous. You can find them on line at www.foodaddicts.org.

Whatever it is, JUST DO IT!!

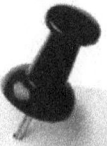

So now the question becomes, "What will you do and to what lengths you are willing to go in order to reach your dream of being thin?"

CHAPTER 16

Enjoying Success with a Reset Hypothalamus

Now that the abnormal excess fat is gone, now what?

If you are like me, you will either be afraid you might gain back the weight, not believe you will, or maybe even decide you worked long and hard enough and now it is time to try it on your own. I know that statistically, most diets fail over time and most dieters regain their lost weight within 1 to 2 years. I understand how this could happen and I am determined not to let it happen to me.

I made my decision early on that since I had spent a lifetime trying so many things without long term success that I was going to continue to follow the "Weight Loss Cure" protocol and guidelines to the best of my ability. I desperately wanted to maintain what I had achieved and not gain back my weight.

I continue to be ecstatic that after doing the protocol twice, following phases 1-4 and then having major cosmetic reconstruction of a large portion of my body (hips, thighs, legs, derriere, and arms), that I have been able to maintain my thin body and not regain my lost weight. Although, I was disappointed that I was not able to stay at my post HCG weight, I am content that I have been able to reach an amazingly slim," normal" body weight that stays consistent within a few pounds range.

I attribute my success to a combination of factors. First, I am sure that there has been a resetting and partial "healing" of my Hypothalamus as a result of taking HCG and following the "Weight Loss Cure" protocol. Second, I have completely accepted that my metabolism was somewhat damaged at an early age from being a fat child and all my "yo-yo dieting". Third, I know that I will ALWAYS need to be very careful what foods I eat and be sure to take in fewer daily calories than what the health/weight guidelines and metabolic formulas tell me.

Lastly and more importantly, I know in my heart that my continued success is directly related to my diligence, consistency and daily continued commitment to myself, my FA program, and following "The Weight Loss Cure" plan. I have faith and honestly believe that if I continue to follow what has been laid out in the "Weight Loss Cure' book and stay Abstinent through my FA recovery program, I will stay slim, healthy and filled with energy and immense joy.

After all I have done to reach my slim body; I want to do everything in my power to retain it and continue to enjoy it. I consider following a plan that works, to be a very small price to pay in order to not return to the past trials and tribulations which once caused me such emotional pain and agony.

I know that as the years go by only time will tell. I can attest to the fact that it has been quite a few years and by following my FA recovery program and my "Weight Loss Cure" regimen, I am still thin, happy, joyous and free and enjoying my body more than I had ever imagined. I still consider it to be quite amazing.

So now the question becomes, "What will you do and to what lengths you are willing to go in order to reach your dream of being thin?" Will you continue to keep trying the latest diet fads out there only to have your efforts fail once again, or will you believe me when I tell you that the "Weight loss Cure" works and go for it yourself?

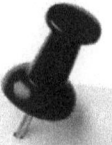

In retrospect, a lot of what had been going on with me was directly related to the effects of my eating sugar and flour products. I also now know that I had some hormonal imbalance going on, that had not been diagnosed.

CHAPTER 17

Thoughts on Mood and Depression

I remember a time when doctors prescribed the medication, Valium, for many women complaining of their monthly menstrual issues of having "moods and "feeling excess stress". In time, after more scientific research and with the experience of understanding, empathetic doctors, many being women, who had actually experienced those same symptoms, PMS was discovered. Another example taken from my own dental profession is the discovery that women have more estrogen receptors in their TMJ apparatus and therefore are more prone to other "stress" responses, including grinding and clenching of their teeth. Over time, science discovers more about the mysteries of our bodies and we get more answers about many that seem troubling to us. These discoveries allow us to live more satisfactory and fulfilling lives.

In my case, I have always felt what I would call "moody" and "melancholic", and I have even gone thru periods that I call "semi-depressed". Somehow, I knew that it was not the type of "depression" that required antidepressant medication in order to function. Most of those times it felt like my body just got out of sync. What I believed and later discovered was that I needed a treatment or "cure" for my undiagnosed, unbalanced, metabolic hormone levels.

I remember clearly the very first time I felt this way and got relief for it. For me, it was actually quite dramatic. In my late twenties, I had begun feeling like there was a dark cloud around me and all my energy seemed to have been zapped out of me. My very skilled therapist referred me to an excellent physician, who found out that I had a thyroid deficiency and needed the thyroid medication, Synthroid.

When I began taking Synthroid, I could not believe how much better I felt. I had immediate relief and felt as if the world had changed around me. I was actually seeing and experiencing the world differently. My energy was back and the dark cloud was gone in a matter of a few days. This doctor explained to me that our hormones control most of the processes going on in our bodies, including our emotions and how we react to stresses in our lives. When they are out of balance or when our endocrine system is not working correctly, it creates havoc in our bodies and problems can occur.

Although I believed my doctor and understood about hormones, I still had some confusion. I had always noticed that when I was thinner, it seemed like I could "control" my moods better and live an easier, happier life. Then, when I would gain weight and was unable to do anything about it, it seemed like I had no control over my mood. My lack of weight control made me feel so powerless and would result in my feeling "depressed". People who I had liked yesterday, I would not like today. I was irritable and "cranky" and became "the great pretender". I would "act" pleasant and want to feel happy, but I was unable to do so.

In retrospect, a lot of what had been going on with me was directly related to the effects of my eating sugar and flour products. I also now know that I had some hormonal imbalance going on, that had not been diagnosed. I remember how difficult it was every day to be constantly fighting so many negative emotions. So much of these mood swings was related to my unexplained weight gains and from the constant cravings and daily struggles with food.

Like most of us, I had been taught that: "calories in equal's calories out". However, I knew my truth was that I seemed to gain weight quicker than everyone else around me and I was unable to find a way to stabilize my slow metabolism. Therefore, I lived with this desperate fear inside of me knowing that I had to eat in order to live, but could not find a way to do so within the bounds of maintaining any stable weight.

Years earlier I had decided that in order to deal with my personal dilemma, I would limit my food intake and eat diet foods, limit external stimuli and stressors and protect myself from the world. I felt I could minimize my inner turmoil by being alone and being as nice to myself as I could. This self-imposed remedy caused me a lot of internal, emotional stress and extreme loneliness. Although this method seemed to work for a short time, eventually my body started regaining excess weight again and a severe melancholy overtook me.

When I had been in FA and abstinent for a while, had NOT had any sugar or flour enter my body for over 7-8yrs, and was still overweight, I once again felt trapped within a gloomy, misty cloud. Feeling betrayed by my body again, I knew I had to search until I found an answer.

What I yearned for and needed was to lose my excess weight, be given "internal sunshine", and be helped to become alive again. There were all kinds of antidepressant medications my various doctors suggested I try, but none of them seemed to help change how I felt or made me feel any better. I knew in my heart that my answer was elsewhere, I just had not found it yet. After reading Dr. Simeone's paper, I knew I had found something worth pursuing. I had the necessary hope that HCG might give me what I was seeking. As you have already read in this book, it definitely has.

One of the things that interested and comforted me the first time I read "The Weight Loss Cure" was the protocol to eat no sugar or flour while following the food plan. I had already been doing this for all my years in FA and it made me feel very comfortable and safe. To me, it seemed the connection to health, metabolic stasis, emotional well-being and weight control might just be found in the "Weight Loss Cure" program in addition to my FA program.

If you are finding yourself battling with mood swings and feel like your emotions are all over the place, take a moment to honestly notice what foods you are putting into your body. If you have the slightest thought that there is a connection for you, be willing to try changing your diet by limiting or stopping your intake of sugar and flour products. Try it for 30 days and notice if you have a clearer mind, more energy and a more positive attitude towards life. This experiment may surprise you and give you an answer you have longed for. If you find a connection, it could change your life for the better. I am sure you will be glad you did.

CHAPTER 18

After Weight Loss

Have you ever noticed how excess weight makes a person look so much older and truly ages a person in body, mind, and spirit? I, myself, felt like a fat, old lady from the time I was in fourth grade until I lost a bulk of my weight and maybe even for a while afterwards. Then when I gained those 27 pounds in 2004, the old feelings that I experienced from when I was a fat, unhappy, little girl in fifth and sixth grade instantly overtook me. There I was once again feeling stuck in a fat woman's body. For me, the fat was imprisoning a beautiful, young girl who felt unable to break out of her prison. It did not matter that the prison was of my own design. I could only watch as my fat body created prejudices about me all over again. I read a quote in a book that said: "fat in our society is the last sanctioned prejudice in our world". That has been my experience, has it been yours?

Since I lost all my weight, so many people tell me how beautiful I look and how much younger I appear to be. I'm told that I can wear anything since it all looks lovely on me. Many of them knew me when I was heavier and they act like it amazes them. As for me, I not only feel prettier, happier, and younger, but I also notice how differently I carry myself. At times, I feel like I actually glide through my day with more confidence and with a little more bounce and energy in my step.

A couple of years ago, I took a writing class and one night the assignment was to remember a time that had emotional impact for us. We had to write the entire story in one-syllable words. The exercise was an eye-opener and surprisingly impactful for me. I want to share it with you, my readers and hopefully by now, my friends. I hope that many of you are considering following "The Weight Loss Cure" for yourself, so you can experience the joy, delight and rewards of being thin, too.

Here is the story I wrote of my childhood memory using only one syllable words:

"I am in eighth grade and school just got out. I go to my desk and get my books to go home. I have a lot to get done. They walk by in twos and threes, but I stand here alone, of course. I think "Why can't I have a friend that stays with me and walks home with me. Can I join Paula? But Paula is so cute, if I could be like her, then they'd like me. I can go to Barb's house when I get home, but I still have to walk home alone. Other kids drive by in cars, but not me. I hope they don't laugh at me or call me names or sing the fat song when they go past. It makes me feel bad and makes me cry. I hate myself. I am so fat. I am so ugly; no one likes me. I walk out the front door and wait so I feel safe. I'll take the small side street so I am alone. Can I hide and not be seen. What do I do if I see the bad kids? I am so afraid they might hurt me. I wish I had someone to help me".

As I was doing the assignment and writing down this memory exercise, I was truly amazed at just how immediate the emotional pain was for me. It was so vivid and so sad that this little ten-year-old child, me, had to experience such terrible pain at such a young age and that it was carried through all the way to my adulthood.

Please do not let this happen to you or your beloved children. Help your children to NOT be fat. Do something now. Help your children to be thinner and healthier and allow them to have the happy childhood they all deserve. Being a child can be difficult enough, they do not need the horrible burden of obesity.

This brings me to the dream I carried inside of me for so many years to just look "normal" to my peers. I have always wanted to just fit in and be accepted by others and not stand out because I looked so distorted. I dreamt constantly of ways to do this and what would happen if I could only one day lose my excess weight.

So, after I had maintained my weight loss for a while and I felt confident that I could keep it off following Phase 4; I started thinking again about getting cosmetic surgery. I kept focusing on the after effects of the weight loss and looking at my areas of aged, sagging skin. I had thought about this before and had even saved some money towards it, but when I had gained the 27 pounds I decided to drop the whole idea. I gave it all up as a hopeless dream.

The only procedure I had considered getting done was to get rid of all the ugly excess skin between my inner thighs. Being very overweight since fourth grade took away most of the firmness and tone from my body. It was the most noticeable in my inner thighs where the skin was extremely stretched out. For many years I was able to ignore the purplish colored stretch marks, since when I lost weight most of them faded to a very light pink in appearance. However, having fat inner thighs and loose, hanging skin meant I had to wear clothes to cover it up, so I would not be afraid to be seen by men that I liked.

When I was a teenager and a young adult trying to date, I tried hard to cover myself up so that I would not experience public embarrassments or attacks on my self-esteem. It was humiliating that when I walked my inner thighs would rub together and chafe and cause severe sores and excruciatingly pain. Not only did I wear out most of my slacks in this area, but trying to function and live normally in the world was severely hampered. I had to find clothes with strong inseams, had to put patches on regularly, and had to constantly monitor myself so I could try to hide the problem. It was such a terrible burden for me to carry around and was a really horrible way for a young woman to grow up.

When I lost weight over the years, I expected that time and exercise would tighten up my sagging skin. However it did not and I was left in a thin body but with debilitating, visible scars, hanging skin and bulges of cellulite. There I was, a woman in my twenties and then thirties who could never wear a bathing suit or shorts without feeling disfigured, when exposing my skin by wearing shorts or a bathing suit. Then as I aged, I not only had loose, hanging skin from weight loss, but also the loss of resiliency and additional sagging from the aging process.

So, you can understand that after my success following "The Weight Loss Cure", I was revisiting the surgery topic once again. Although, there was no guarantee as to just how long I could keep my weight stable, I made a promise to myself that I would never again be fat and I would do whatever it took for me to be thin. I wanted to keep my slim shape and newly found joy. As I wrote earlier, for a time I thought it meant that I would have to follow a weekly, Phase 4, diet steak day, but I was entirely willing to do so. It really seemed like such a small price to pay for what I had achieved. The only issue I felt I had left was how to get rid of the loose skin between my inner thighs.

At times, I would think that maybe I was too old and "past my prime" to have cosmetic surgery, and I would tell myself that it was not worth it. However, I knew in my heart of hearts that I just had to do it. The purpose for the surgery was not only to help improve my physical appearance, but also to help me complete my thinning out process. I also fully believed that it would allow my self-esteem to increase in a way it never could have before. I hoped it would aid to complete the healing process of that little; helpless, fat child that still resided within me. I do not think we ever totally outgrow or forget our childhood wounds which settle so deep in our souls at such a tender age. However, I believe that we can definitely take actions to minimize the effects our past still has on us.

Ultimately, I decided that I was ready and could go through cosmetic surgery. I imagined that it could be a very emotional process for me, and I expected that after the healing period, I would not only look and feel better, but I would be healed from some of the past emotional and spiritual scars. I thought about how I could eventually share my personal experiences in order to help another "prior fat child" make decisions about their adult, sagging skin or perhaps, even help prevent them from ever even going through any of it.

One of the reasons I am so adamant about sharing my life with you and what keeps me so highly motivated, is what I see happening all around me. Currently in our society there is just so much obesity of children at younger and younger ages. I read about the horrible abuse of bullying by youngsters' peers, and how our newer technologies can cause incredible pain and devastation in children's lives. I pray that maybe I can make even a small, positive impact for at least a few of them, to not have to go through my ordeal and painful experiences. One of my desires in writing this book is that if at least one child's life will be improved then that would make all that I have been through a really worthwhile journey.

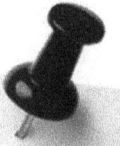

This first look into what the surgical consequences would be for me stopped me from going any further, until more time had passed and I was really ready to go forward.

CHAPTER 19

Cosmetic Surgery: The Why, How and the Process

For a long, long time, I had pre-diagnosed my body's reconstructive needs and determined what I thought would "fix" my problems. Having been fat, since I was 10 years old and having lost and gained weight so many times over the years, I could see that I had lost most of the elasticity of the skin on my hips, thighs and middle third of my body. I was burdened with dark, purple-red, stretch marks on many visible parts of my body. Whether I wore sleeveless shirts, shorts or bathing suits, not only could you see my excess fat, but also numerous, red, stretch marks that were the kind commonly seen in pregnant women. Needless to say, these ugly stretch marks on my young girl's body were not only unsightly, but also a cause for my intense embarrassment and shame.

Even when I covered my body with slacks, I inevitably wore through the material at the inner thigh areas, requiring my mother to place "patches" in order to extend the longevity of my clothing. It never mattered what type of pants she'd buy for me, they always wore through and needed repair. When I would try to wear a dress or a pair of shorts, my thighs would chafe and become red and lead to raw sores that made it too painful to walk. I have many memories of having to wear a panty girdle or stockings with a garter belt when I was only an 11or 12 year old girl. Not only was it painful and debilitating, physically, but it also forced me to accept just how different I was from my "peers" and to try to keep myself "invisible' or hidden as much as I could. I did this by not accepting invitations, when I got them, and meticulously planning just how I could hide my body from others judgment and ridicule.

Can you just imagine what kind of terrible burden this caused for a prepubescent, young girl? I carried around the feeling of being different for many years. When I began my research into cosmetic surgery in 1999, and a kind friend who used to be very obese took me into the ladies room to show me her surgical scars, I was fascinated that there was no hanging flesh or many visible stretch marks.

It is no small statement when I say that I was shocked and somewhat scared off, when she showed me her circumferential scarring across the entire ½ of her body. It looked like someone had painted on a bikini scar line around her. It caused me to have a flashback to a horror movie I had once seen, where someone's head was cut off and then they were cut in half at the waist. It was a very gruesome thought, but so was someone allowing anyone to carve you up with a knife, by choice!

This first look into what the surgical consequences would be for me stopped me from going any further, until more time had passed and I was really ready to go forward.

However, I did continue to imagine what it would be like to actually walk around without my inner thighs rubbing together and I dreamed what it would feel like to wear a dress without nylon stockings. Since I was obviously not ready to undergo any type of reconstructive surgery, I decided to put this entire surgery idea out of my head until I had lost ALL of my excess weight. I felt that at the appropriate time, I could re-visit the possibility of my having cosmetic surgery.

As more weight came off, around the years 2000-2001, I did notice my flesh becoming looser and hanging even more, especially along my inner thighs. I began to reconsider the surgical idea and I went for 3 surgical consultations. This started my pre-research into what type of re-contouring my body actually needed to give my inner thighs the "normal" contour I so desired.

Then, over the next few years, I kept struggling with getting off the last 20 excess pounds, and my metabolism issues resurfaced as my body responded to Perimenopause and Menopause. This was when I regained almost 27 pounds and no one was able to explain the cause of the weight gain or help me do anything about it. I became so upset and stressed by my ever-widening body, that the idea of cosmetic surgery seemed ludicrous.

The major change for me came after I found HCG and "The Weight Loss Cure" Program and I found the way to finally take off my excess weight and rid my body of all the "abnormal fat stores". The thin body I was left with after following "The Weight loss Cure" program, felt like such a gift and what I called a true miracle. It was then, that I began to truly fanaticize what it would be like if my body, most specifically, my inner thighs, could be reshaped to give me the appearance and function of "normal looking' legs.

Now the idea of noticeable scarring didn't worry me as much as it had previously. I think that was due to my getting used to showing these glaring, visible, purple-red or fading pink stretch marks, since I was ten. I had reached a point when I felt I just wanted to get rid of the excess skin. As I look back, I also believe that I could not fully fathom what it would be like to have actual scars on my body, and I minimized to myself what it would feel like seeing them every day.

Now that I have the luxury of hindsight and can appreciate my journey in retrospect, I can see what I should have done differently and wished I had known.

It is important that you understand that once you have any kind of surgery, you WILL be different. Your body has been forever altered and in some way it will change your world, and how you function within it. Surgery of any type is an assault on the body; even though you may have fully planned it. It can be considered an injury of some type, to the creation by God, which is you. It's important to plan for and expect this change and know that it may NOT end up "exactly" as you wanted or expected.

The hope in most of us is that the change will give us what we desire, be an improvement and positive result, and that our joy will be instantaneous. However you must remember to always keep your expectations realistic and accept that there will most likely be some price to pay. That price might be the long healing time, amount of soreness you experience, excessive time off from work, inability to carry on your normal routine, change in your physical movement, unexpected aches or muscle changes from your change in gait and the list goes on.

The surgeons give out a list on possible side effects that are related to the physical possibilities. However, they do not give out or have any realistic way of suggesting or predicting what type of emotional or spiritual effects it will have on you. Of course, even if they could offer a potential list, so much depends on your individual past history; including personal experiences and events you have lived thru, your individual personality, your desires, hopes, dreams and expectations, and how your own body will neurologically and biochemically be affected by the specific surgical trauma you have undergone.

Sometimes, even the most well thought out and desired plan can turn out totally different than you imagined. If you question this at all, just read any of the popular magazines, discussing the movie stars and their cosmetic surgery stories.

It's not unusual for former fat women and men to undertake cosmetic surgery after losing their excess weight. Once the fat is gone, the previously fat person is left with areas of loose, hanging skin that is not only unsightly, but also annoying and a constant reminder of the prior fat condition they were in for so long. Depending on just how long one has been fat, there is the added burden of overstretched skin, stretch marks, and a loss of much of the skin's elasticity, which normal skin would have.

Each individual must decide for themselves if surgery is the appropriate path for them. Some people look older and haggard, due to the loss of excess fat from their face and neck, others have excess skin layers hanging off their arms, legs, thighs or midriff and still others have the sagging skin around their stomach or buttocks. Depending on where the excess skin is located, there are a multitude of surgical corrective procedures that can be done to remove the offensive skin and "tighten up" the areas needing re-contouring. Most if not all of these procedures require much forethought including: planning, budgeting of time, money and resources for research and surgical consultations and then treatment. Ultimately, the "decision of choice" is whether to have surgery or not.

One must determine for oneself, if they want to go "under the knife" with general anesthesia and all that it entails, or whether to live with the consequences and "battle scars", of one's previously obese condition, and learn to accept oneself as they are. The operative question becomes; "Can you find a way to overlook the sagging flesh and prepare yourself as it worsens with age and the effects of gravity or not?"

My Process: Before, During and After

For me, the decision process was a very lengthy one. I first began thinking about having "liposuction" after my 1st really big weight loss. I watched a 60 Minutes show on liposuction and saw a woman's "before and after" photos. The change in this woman's stomach and outer thighs and body shape was nothing short of amazing. I began to wonder if what she had undergone would give me the same results.

Then in 1999, I met with a woman who had liposuction and extensive cosmetic surgery along her thighs and entire circumference of her lower body. She told me she was pleased with her results for the most part and said she was glad she did it and would do it over again. She said her surgery had changed the way she viewed herself and how she related in the world.

At the time, I thought I could keep it simple and just have Liposuction and not need any surgical intervention. I definitely didn't think I would need the type of extensive surgery this woman had to have. I researched all about liposuction and what it would entail and found so many negative outcomes listed and possible side effects, that I became extremely worried and decided not to do anything.

Then over time as I lost and regained my weight, I noticed that my skin was sagging more and more and I began to consider that I may actually need surgery to correct it. As I allowed this idea to sink into my mind, I began wondering what really could be done with my inner thighs to make them look normal. I read articles on different types of cosmetic surgery and realized I might actually need to have a "lower body lift" surgery to give me the result I wanted. Being very afraid of having any type of surgery done to my body, I did nothing for a long time. I just waited and kept thinking about what I might look like if and when I decided to get something done.

I actually thought about having cosmetic surgery, specifically the lower body lift, for almost eight years before I did the intensive research into actually having it done. I then spent two additional years consulting with cosmetic surgeons, reviewing the possible pros and cons and consequences, and talking with women that had gone thru the process. When I finally decided to plan and actually have it done, I spent another year consulting with the surgeon I chose, and determining if I wanted all the four/five suggested surgeries done together, what it would actually mean to me emotionally, physically, and spiritually, in addition to how it would affect my ability to work and my home life.

As I look back now and give consideration to all my preplanning, I see that I was still totally unprepared for the process that followed, especially the amount of healing time I would need and the repercussions it would have on all the other systems in my body. Post-surgery, I felt totally taken by surprise when I realized I was having deleterious side effects felt by my stomach and GI system, my musculoskeletal system, especially my neck and back, and the change in my mobility of how I moved about in the world. It has most definitely affected my work life, my social and personal life, and my home life and marriage. At times I have even felt "disabled" and "traumatized" by it all.

And remember dear readers, I "wanted" this surgery, truly believed it was in my best interest to do all of it, at one time, that it would offer me the dreams I had hoped for, and that it would only affect my future in a very positive way. I thought it would help put closure on and help heal my troubled childhood and that feel beautiful, happier and more secure in my body. I imagined that I would be able to walk and sway with more grace and sensuality, allowing me to become sexier.

So what a shock it was to me, when immediately afterwards, I became hunched over, had pain in my back, could barely walk by myself and could NOT enjoy my new svelte shape and even began to feel like a little old woman. For me to continue to have to sleep with pillows propping me up for support, and still be numb throughout my mid-body many years later, was never once a consideration or thought in my head.

Fortunately, I never stopped looking for answers and have developed an excellent network of practitioners and alternative healers. They have helped me improve some of the more troublesome consequences of the surgery, so I have been able to enjoy my new body and move forward in my life.

However, given all the unexpected side issues that my surgery has created for me, I need to say that I still have thoroughly enjoyed having no hanging excess skin, having a firm, svelte body and being able to buy clothes that fit snugly and show off my amazing shape. I can also honestly say that it has helped improve my self-esteem and body image and repair some of my long standing, emotional childhood wounds.

CHAPTER 20

Choosing a Cosmetic Surgeon

As I have already said, I had done extensive research and consulted with many cosmetic surgeons before finding the one that fit all my necessary criteria. I needed to know that they had a good reputation and were very skilled in the specific surgeries I needed done. I also had to feel completely comfortable in their bedside manner and treatment of me and if possible, I wanted them to be located within a reasonable travel distance. It seemed to be an important consideration that their office was close to my home, if possible, since I knew there would be pre-surgical consultations and many post-operative appointments.

When I had first considered having any treatment at all, I went to a local cosmetic surgeon who told me I was a candidate for liposuction, but I would also need a "lower body lift" in order to achieve what I wanted. I was pretty overwhelmed and did not feel comfortable with him and what he explained about the surgical process, so I decided to hold off until I thought about it some more.

It was about six months later when a physician I knew referred me to a well-respected surgical team in Boston. When I went for my consultation, I liked the surgeons, but their office seemed extremely disorganized. Then the few times I called their office, there had either been a change of staff or no one returned my calls. I questioned whether the unstable staff and poor office organization was a reflection on the surgeons and I decided to start looking elsewhere.

I then checked our local yellow pages and did an internet search and came up with a few names. One doctor had so many degrees and training that I thought he might be the one. So, I called his office to schedule a preliminary consultation. I told the receptionist that I was considering a "lower body lift" to get rid of all the ugly sagging skin on my inner thighs that had limited me all my life, and I wanted an appointment to meet the doctor and staff, ask some general questions, get an evaluation of what I wanted looked at and find out if I could have it done. I shared with her that I just wanted my legs to look "normal".

When I was speaking with her, I kept thinking that for as long as I could remember, starting back in junior high school I watched the skin on my inner thighs keep sagging and only getting worse over time. Then as I became an older, more "mature" woman and with all my excess body weight gone via HCG, I could actually see how much sagging and excess skin there really was. I had also begun to notice that my upper, inner arms, my rear end, and my back outer thighs had more sagging skin that I hadn't noticed before.

I expected to schedule a brief appointment with the surgeon and then either move forward or keep searching. Well, what a surprise it was when I wasn't even allowed to schedule a consult with the doctor. After four phone calls, the receptionist told me that I would have to have a full series of medical tests and a referral from my family doctor proving that I was healthy, before her doctor would give permission for me to come in for a consult. She actually said that her doctor's time was extremely important and could not be "wasted" on "just" a consult with me, which might not lead to his accepting me as a patient.

Well, at first I became quite outraged, but then I thought: "Why would I ever want this judgmental, egomaniac for a doctor?" Then I began to wonder if he had been involved in some poor outcome cases and was protecting himself. Neither of these thoughts made me feel comfortable going to him for anything, especially to cut on my precious body.

I knew I wanted a skilled surgeon, but I also wanted a human being with some humility and one that I could trust to treat me well. I had dreamt about this surgery for many years and I needed to feel safe, secure and totally comfortable with the surgeon I chose.

It was suggested that I keep asking for referrals from people that had undergone cosmetic surgery. I connected with a woman who had lost 180 pounds and had gone through many surgeries to remove her excess skin and contour her body. She raved about how wonderful her surgeon was, gave me his name, and told me she "trusted him with her life".

She convinced me that he would treat me well and I would have an excellent result. So I made an appointment for a consult, and had my husband, Curt, accompany me for support and as an objective resource. When I make up my mind to do something, I usually do not need anyone else as a backup. However, I wanted my husband's honest opinion about something this major. I knew that a surgery of this magnitude could be potentially dangerous and life changing. I realized that I would want Curt's full support before, during and after the actual surgery.

Well, my first impression of the office was that everyone was kind and professional and knew what they were doing. It was interesting, though; that during the initial examination with the doctor, I felt that he was too clinical and did not possess the warm bedside manner I wanted or had seen in all his staff.

After my exam, the doctor came back to talk with us, and he seemed a bit more relaxed and willing to answer the many questions I asked. He gave me all the time I needed and never shut me up or tried to push me along. He pointed out a few things I was not fully aware of and showed how the sagging that I thought involved only my inner thighs and inner upper arms actually extended along my midriff, my stomach, my rear end and back thigh area. I had never realized that it was all sagging skin from weight loss. He pointed out those areas where I had most recently lost additional weight during the HCG process, losing what we call cellulite. I actually thought that I still had some remaining fat, but he assured me that all my fat was gone.

I had so much stretched out and distorted skin from when I was ten years old, that the sagging was actually a result of my skin's inability to tighten up. He compared my skin to an elastic band that has been stretched out too much, and told me my skin would never firm up on its own. My body would require surgical intervention if I wanted to get rid of the excess skin. His diagnosis did not surprise me in the least.

I also asked him some of my other questions. I wanted to know about some of the different types of surgeries available, what type would give me the final results I wanted, how much time I would be in the operating room, how long would I be under General Anesthesia, what were the possible complications, who would be involved in my surgery, who would be allowed in the operating room, how long I would be off from work and what the total cost would be. I think I have watched too many hospital TV shows and listened to too many horror stories about patients in hospitals where bad things happened. I did not want any interns or residents in my operating room "learning" on me or touching me.

He answered all my questions and told me he had his own surgical team and hospital anesthesiologist who worked with him. He assured me that he could help me and remove the sagging skin from my inner thighs, so they would finally not chafe when I walk and not be unsightly no matter what I wore. He assured me that I would be extremely satisfied with the result and I felt confident that I was in the right office.

However, the treatment would be much more extensive than I had thought, and there would be many surgical scars as a result. The cost would also be a lot more than I had originally budgeted for. As I considered what he had told me, I realized that I was now seven years older than when I had first thought seriously about having it done and I had even regained some weight, one more time. I had followed the HCG treatment procedures and I had finally loss <u>all my excess fat</u>.

He pointed out what he could do for me, that it would involve 4 to 5 surgeries, gave me the estimated fees, and then informed me that I could even have it all done at the same time. He said if I did so, then some of the fees would be reduced, since I was already in the operating room. Although I was skeptical, he assured me that he could do it all at one time and told me that it would require a full day of surgery with general anesthesia.

I had to accept that the result of all my yo-yoing with dieting was having lots of sagging skin. I liked this doctor and his office, but felt that I still needed some time to process all the information I had just learned. So, I decided I would consider scheduling a second consult for him to show me some actual before and after photos, and answer any additional questions. The receptionist suggested I schedule a surgery date, but I told her I needed time to read the brochures and I would call in a week or so to talk about surgery dates.

I left his office knowing that I needed some time to process what he had said and whether I was going to be able to go thru with it. I felt both excited and extremely anxious. There was just so much to think about. Was I really ready to have someone cut up my body? Would it be worth it? Would I mind the scarring? Was it worth the possible risk of having a reaction to the General Anesthesia and possibly even death? I knew that death from this type of surgery was a rare occurrence, but I still had to consider it as a possibility.

I considered how ludicrous it was that I had spent my entire life protecting my body from any physical injury, never breaking anything and never taking undo risks that could cause me to end up in a hospital requiring any type of surgery. Yet, here I was actually considering going into a hospital by choice and having surgery done.

The next two weeks, I was obsessed with the whole surgery process. I could not get my mind off of it. I began working out the exact specifics that I knew would determine my final decision. I thought that I would have to block off a minimum of three and a half to four weeks from my practice and considered all the logistics that would entail. At the time, I wouldn't allow myself to consider that I could take off any more time, due to the financial hardship I felt it would create for me.

I continued to do more research, read more specific articles on my four possibly 5 surgeries, spoke with friends and met again with those who had undertaken my type of surgery, so I could view their scars. I really wanted to go thru with it, but I was still hesitating and undecided. My friends told me their specific suggestions and were very willing to show me and discuss their scarring. Most of what they showed me did not bother me as much as I had expected.

My reservations were not only taking time off from work and getting coverage, but also getting the finances in order to do it. I was also overwhelmed by how much surgery it would entail and whether I should do only the lower body lift or should I just get it all done at one time. However, the more I thought about it the more doable it became for me. I spoke again to my friend that had had all the surgeries and got her reassurance about the doctor and her assessment that it was the best thing she had ever done. She told me that the result of her surgeries had impacted her life for the better and that if I could afford it all I should just get it done.

So in the next few weeks, I sat with my husband and reviewed what the surgeon had said, talked about my concerns, pondered and read the brochures over and over again, and got excited waiting for the next consult. I could only imagine what the surgery would be like and what it would do for me. I wondered if it would really make a difference and would it do for me what I had hoped for.

My husband told me to "go for it" and said that he backed me one hundred percent. When I began finding objections and voicing my doubts saying comments like: "maybe I am too old", his response was, "I think it is the next important step for you to complete the process of all the hard work you have done!" I knew in my heart, that he was right. This surgery on my inner thighs was important for my self-esteem, to be able to move on from regretting and mourning my past, and for my functioning better physically. Knowing Curt was fully supportive of my decision allowed me to start becoming even more excited about the final result.

As I considered having all five surgeries done, I realized one aspect that really concerned me was the inner arm scarring, since that would be the most noticeable of all. I had to honestly ask myself, just how badly I disliked my sagging upper arms. Was it enough to warrant a noticeable scar forever? That's when I realized that I definitely needed to go for another consult to see more photos to help me finalize my surgical decision and ask those nagging, gut wrenching questions that still kept me afraid and uncertain.

So, over the next few months, I went for 2 more surgical consultations. These appointments turned out to be very important for me. At each one I looked at many before and after photos of the doctor's patients, showing all the surgeries I was considering, especially the upper arms. I was fascinated with the changes in people's bodies after their surgeries, but noticed how they all had quite a bit of scarring. When I voiced this concern, the doctor told me the scarring from the tummy tuck and derriere lift surgeries could be covered by a bikini bottom. However, the lower thigh lift would show some scarring along my inner leg and the arm lift surgery could be very visible, depending how far down he would have to go to get a nice clean line.

He said the surgery would remove all the sagging skin and assured me that my final result would look good, but that I would have to decide if I wanted to live with the unsightly, sagging skin that I came in with or accept the resulting purplish scarring afterwards. He said that the scarring would appear reddish-purple after the surgery and would lighten up to a deep pink over time and be much less noticeable. He suggested that I take time to consider all the pros and cons involved and decide what surgeries I wanted to have done. He advised me to schedule a definite surgery date and then sent me home with the pre-operative instructions and all the necessary paperwork for my upcoming surgery.

The surgeon and his entire staff were wonderful. I had pretty much decided I would have four of the surgeries done for sure and probably also the fifth, upper arm surgery. We discussed the length of the surgery and reviewed how the hospital stay would work. He suggested I plan on staying at least 1 night at the hospital and I decided I would stay 2 nights, knowing that I was going to have a lot of surgery and would most likely need the extra night. I was also considering my husband, who would be my full time caretaker, and would have his hands full nursing me into recovery. I felt we would both be more comfortable if I stayed two nights having skilled nursing care helping me.

Being anxious to get the process started and with the receptionist's urging, I scheduled the pre-operative surgical consultation with his receptionist and a possible surgery date. Although I was excited, I surprisingly left the office feeling even more doubts than I had come in with. I knew I wanted to get rid of the excess skin, but I feared how bad my body would look with all the scarring.

However, after much more thought, I decided to move forward and go for it all. I chose to have all of the surgeries done at one time and accept that I would have some scarring, but be grateful that all my hanging skin would be gone. I imagined that I would look at my body and there would be no unsightly flesh hanging. I would be able to walk around without stockings and feel comfortable and happy. I was ready!

I never had any serious reservations about whether I would be able to function after all the healing was done. My doctor told me it would be optimum if I took off between 4-6 weeks from work, but a minimum of three and a half weeks was mandatory and would probably be sufficient. He also added that my body would need time to be stretched out and recuperate from all the surgery. It would take approximately 12-18 months before all the numbness would be gone and I would function like before.

We decided that I would return to work after 4 weeks post-surgery, doing light activities at first and slowly resume my normal work schedule. My surgeon never once indicated that I would not heal as expected or that I would have any unforeseen issues or problems.

It still surprises me that with all my research and preparation that I was completely taken off guard and blind sighted by just how debilitated I became and how vulnerable and helpless I felt post operatively. I had never experienced anything like that before and hope to never have to feel that way again!

CHAPTER 21

Key Journal Notes Regarding My Surgical Experience

Tuesday, August 19th

Today I went for my final consult with the cosmetic surgeon. I asked my final list of questions, reviewed what the protocol was, got all my medications, and had my body marked up in ink in preparation for the all-day surgery the following day, Wednesday, 8/20/08.

Author's Note: *Looking back now, it amazes me that I could have asked so many questions and read so much about the surgical process, and still have been somewhat clueless and poorly informed about what to expect afterwards and just how it would actually impact my life.*

Wednesday, August 20th
My Surgery Day

I reported in at 6:15am to the Surgical Center of Cape Cod Hospital. I checked in, filled out the required paperwork, was taken into a dressing room, and told to put on a hospital gown and surgical clothes. Looking back now, it all seemed a bit surreal at the time.

I was told to lie down on a surgical table, asked a lot of questions, and had an IV line put into my right arm. Then I was visited by a nurse, a counselor, an anesthesiologist, my Plastic Surgeon and his surgical nurse. I know I was transferred onto an operating room transfer table, but I really can't remember much more about what went on after that, because my pre-surgical medications had begun to kick in. I do remember feeling somewhat anxious about the upcoming operation and at the same time calm and almost resigned to the entire event. Fortunately, I do not remember anything about the OR suite, the anesthesia or what happened during the actual surgery.

The next thing I remember is waking up in a hospital bed with my husband alongside me. When I opened my eyes, I could tell I was lying down and felt woozy and barely able to move. A nurse told me I was in a corner suite of the Cape Cod Pediatric unit and had been transferred there from the recovery room. I noticed that I was covered by a sheet, and was told that I had 6 drains attached to me and a special black box around my neck that released small amounts of the anesthetic, Lidocaine.

I glanced around the room and saw a bouquet of flowers on a table to my left and my husband anxiously watching me. I had absolutely no memory of the operating room or the recovery room or how I got into that bed. I felt extremely "off", had nausea, felt pain all over my body and my throat hurt a lot. I remember that I could feel vibrators on both of my lower legs.

The nurse told me I had a catheter in, that the surgery had gone well and offered me pain medication. My choices were Morphine, IV Demerol or Darvocet. Being in such pain and unable to think clearly, I asked my husband his suggestion and requested the Demerol.

I remember getting the Demerol shot and a heparin shot, and my lower legs being massaged and then I was out until Thursday AM, when my surgeon came in and talked to me. That entire Thursday I felt like I was in a daze, kind of like I was outside myself looking in, and I felt very spacey and "out of it'. I was offered food, but I could barely eat anything until Friday.

They took out my catheter either late Thursday or Friday morning and told me I had to get up and go to the bathroom. I was in a lot of pain, felt dizzy and extremely nauseous. I had never experienced anything like that before. I did not want to move. The nurse told me that I would have to get up and start walking. I remember hearing the words and thinking, "she's got to be crazy, I'm not going anywhere!"

When I was finally more alert and could focus on more than my intense pain, I looked around and saw that I was in a lovely suite at the end of a pediatric unit. There was even a nice cot in the corner by the window for my husband to stay at night. I did not expect him to stay with me, but having the cot there was very comforting and gave me a feeling of additional safety knowing he could be close by, looking out for me. My husband did decide to stay with me the entire time and sleep in the cot until I was discharged. As I look back, I can see that as hard as it all was for me, it was the best situation possible, and I am glad it worked out as well as it did.

The nurses told me that they had been giving me regular heparin shots, so I would not develop blood clots. They also kept my legs vibrating constantly to keep the circulation flowing in my legs. Although it felt odd, it did give me a sense of well-being and safety. The nursing care was superb and I realized as I began to come around more and was moved from the bed to the bathroom, that I needed a lot more time to adjust to my post-surgery state.

Friday, August 22nd

When my surgeon came in on Friday and told me I was scheduled to leave later that day, I told him there was no way I was going anywhere. I told him I HAD to stay another day. He told me that was fine with him. He said that he would not discharge me until I was ready, but it would cost me another night's charge. I remember thinking that after all the money I had already spent for my surgery another night's stay was the least of my concerns. I knew I could not get up out of bed by myself or get out and walk, and I certainly could not get into a car to be driven home. As it turned out, the $250 per night cost for the room was well worth it, since I had supervised nursing care and constant attention.

In retrospect my original idea to only stay 1 extra night in order to have skilled nursing care was extremely naïve on my part. There was just so much I did not realize about how debilitated, helpless and needy I would be, until after I was already laid up in the hospital. I could barely move or get up to even use the bathroom without lots of outside help, and I knew that only staying 2 days and nights would not be enough.

I had been in the operating room for a total of 7 and ½ hours under General Anesthesia and I had several separate surgeries done. Let me tell you exactly what that entailed. I had a "Lower Body Lift" including a" Thigh Lift", a "Derriere Lift", a "Tummy Tuck" and an "Arm Lift", or Brachioplasty. When I had decided to do all of these surgeries together in one long operation, I had believed that doing it this way, instead of being in the OR under General anesthesia 2-3 separate times, made a lot of sense and would let me get it all done and over with. I thought my body would heal up simultaneously, need less time off of work and would keep me from experiencing excessive post-operative problems. However, if I were to go back in time and do it all over again, I most assuredly would have done it differently. I have discovered that for me it was way too much surgery being done at one time.

My surgeon told me he had removed 3.8 pounds of skin from my body and that I had absolutely No fat to be removed, only skin. Let me say here to all my readers that I had never expected to hear those words from anyone, least of all a doctor. Most of my prior doctors had suggested diets to me or tried to reassure me that having "some extra weight" on my body was not the worst thing I could have. So after my surgeon told me about having no fat to be removed, all I could think of was that it was all a result of my successfully following the HCG "Weight Loss Cure" program.

My surgeon then told me he would see me the next morning on Saturday to release me from the hospital and approved my staying over another night. The nurses taking care of me were extremely attentive and kind. So when my day nurse told me very firmly that if I stayed over this additional night, I had to get up and walk 3 times on Friday in order to leave on Saturday, I knew she meant it. However, I had no idea how I was going to be able to do it whether she expected it or not.

I have to stress to all my readers that just going to the bathroom was so very hard for me. It took all the energy I could muster, made me feel dizzy and nauseous, and hurt like hell. I felt like I was one big bruise. My entire body ached and cried out in pain. Since it was such a huge ordeal for me to get up and go to the bathroom, I tried hard not to go. However, as the saying goes: When you've got to go, you've got to go.

My post-surgery discomfort and my inability to move by myself were so extreme, that it was very wise for me to stay the 3 full days and nights at the hospital. It allowed me just enough time to begin recuperating, while allowing the skilled nurses to care for me and prepare me for how it would be after I left the hospital.

The entire process was so much more than I imagined and what I could have ever anticipated. I'm so glad that I just accepted that I needed the nursing care and did not allow myself to feel guilty or worried about the additional cost.

In order to be prepared to be discharged from the hospital, the nurses had to teach us how to take care of all my drains, dress my incisions and do all it would take to help my post-operative recovery. I had hired a friend, who was a health care aid, who would come in daily to relieve my loving husband for a few hours a day, and to also be trained how to care for me once I was discharged. Getting up and moving around was such an ordeal, because in addition to my having to somehow lift myself up off the bed, I also had to carry around the 6 drains and the "Big Black Box". I felt like a cow wearing a cow bell! Perhaps, to an observer, I even looked like one.

Saturday, August 23rd

On Saturday, late morning, after my surgeon discharged me, I was helped into a wheelchair, and taken to our car by my husband. It took a lot of effort and assistance to lift me into our car's passenger seat and lay the chair back, so I could be somewhat comfortable. I slept until we got home, where Curt was able to lift me all by himself and eventually guide me into the house and onto the recliner section at the end of the sofa. Although, normally our recliner can be quite comfy, I found it to be extremely uncomfortable. My entire body just hurt, no matter what position I was in.

As I was trying to rest in our recliner, I realized that I was hungry. I had eaten very little while in the hospital, even though I had brought all my weighed and measured food with me. At the hospital, I had been lying down the entire time and feeling nauseous and in too much pain to eat. My throat had ached from the intubation tube that was down my throat for the 7 and ½ hour surgery. The result of the tube being in for so long was a very sore throat and too much pain for me to swallow. It also left me sounding quite funny for about 4 days. My throat healed rather quickly and felt much better by late Saturday, allowing me to resume a very limited, soft eating plan.

Most of my memories from that Saturday and Sunday are pretty much a blur. I do remember that the sofa's recliner turned out to be too uncomfortable for me to stay in. My husband had to call our handyman, and together they brought our comfortable, old, blue leather lounge recliner up from the basement for me to use. This became my bed and place of refuge for the next 4 weeks. It was still a challenge to get comfortable, but thank goodness we had it. It made the entire recuperation process bearable.

As I already mentioned, I had hired a health care worker to help me out once I was home. This friend was a CNA, but she seemed insecure and confused about how to deal with my drains. In retrospect, I believe she was over her head in how to care for someone after such extensive surgery. However, she did try her best and was a support for both me and my husband.

My husband was absolutely wonderful and took on the full responsibility of my nursing care. Thank goodness he understood about how the drains worked, was strong enough to lift me up and take care of me, and took care of the furniture moving required for my post-surgical care. I advise anyone planning for major cosmetic surgery to arrange to have a full time caregiver lined up for their post-surgical care.

What did I have to deal with? I had 6 drains hanging off of my body. One on the right thigh, one on the left thigh, one on my right rear, one on my left rear, one on my right front abdomen and one on my left front abdomen. In addition, I had a specially ordered large, square, "Black Box" that hung off of my neck. This box was a "Pain Pump" that dispensed Lidocaine directly into my abdominal incision to keep it numb and allow me to use less Percocet and Vicodin for pain. I'm sure it helped a lot and I recommend anyone undergoing my type of surgery to ask about it.

However, you must remember that it is one more thing hanging off your body and will quickly become cumbersome and annoying. It also limits movement when repositioning yourself and going to the bathroom. I am uncertain if I would order the "Black Box" again. When I was in my post-operative phase, I had to keep telling myself that it was keeping the pain down and that the annoyance was worth it.

Over the Following Weeks

Over the next week I was able to adapt and somehow settle into the blue leather rocker-recliner as my bed. I never could have adjusted without the constant and tender care from my loving husband. He developed a way to help me sit down, then lift me up and slide me back towards the chair, all the while protecting my arms from getting damaged. Then he would envelop me in pillows to help my sore, ravaged body be as comfortable as possible. I say the word comfortable very hesitantly, because I really was never anything like comfortable for the first 4 weeks.

For the first 2 weeks, following my surgeon's instructions, I kept on track with my Percocet and other medications in order keep the pain from getting ahead of me. I slept whenever possible; listened to healing tapes I had made prior to the surgery, and did a lot of meditation. I also listened to Books on Tape as a distraction and as a way to pass the time. Since I had also had both of my arms surgically altered, I could not hold my hands up to read a book or do any writing. I was truly incapacitated.

As I look back over the entire process, I am sure you can appreciate why I thought that I looked like a skinned chicken. I was cut along my upper inner legs, along my inner thighs, under my stomach and along my lower back, around the back of my upper legs and along the inner section of my upper arms.

I cannot clearly remember much of my day to day doings for the first week or two. What I do remember is having my husband and my health aid caring for me and moving me from chair to bathroom, draining my drains, giving me food when I could eat, dispensing needed drugs and checking on me a lot. As I said above, I spent most of my time trying to sleep and meditate on healing so I would not feel the pain.

One of the most traumatic events, I remember, occurred very early on. My health aid was caring for me, while my husband was working upstairs. I asked her to help get me up and take me to the bathroom. As she tried to help me get up, she somehow forgot about my arm surgery and she dug her fingers into the surgical area of my right inner arm. I remember screaming in pain and almost falling down until my husband ran from upstairs and took over and laid me down. This injury kept my right inner arm in pain much longer than my left and definitely slowed down the healing process. I realized then that although my friend was doing the best she could, that she was not really trained for my post-operative care as I had hoped.

You can see why I feel it necessary to warn you to be sure to get yourself a well-trained caretaker to help you BEFORE you undergo any major surgery. We each must be our own health care advocate. We will be the ones affected and are therefore ultimately responsible for the choices we make. I had assumed that her having CNA training would fully prepare her for my needs, but I was wrong. This incident taught me to ask more specific questions and never to assume anything of anybody.

Another incident occurred on the Monday following my surgery. After being home for 3 days, I asked my husband to lift me up and walk me to the bathroom. I remember that I felt weak and a bit faint and saying so. The next thing I remembered was falling onto the hard bathroom floor and when I awoke, I was on the den floor with bleeding from my inner arm. I heard my husband saying that I was "bleeding like a stuck pig" and "I would be all right". I saw the blood on the kitchen floor and the den carpet and became even fainter. He put a big towel under my right arm and told me to stay put while he went to clean up the bloody mess from the bathroom to the den. That entire event was terrifying for me. After he cleaned things up, he helped me back into the recliner and I fell asleep. When I awoke, he was beside me, checking my right arm and telling me I would be fine.

Thank goodness those were the only two traumatic events that happened after I got home. I am very grateful that much of those first two weeks post-surgery is just a blur to me now. I know that friends came to visit, brought flowers and gifts and said they would be in touch. I remember feeling extremely cared about and loved and extremely grateful for the friends I had. People did such kind things for me and it made me wonder why it seems to take a tragedy or a difficult time for us to notice how cared about we are.

Tuesday was my first big excursion since the surgery. I had to go for a follow up appointment with my surgeon in Hyannis. It was such a challenge to get out of the recliner at home, have Curt place me into the passenger seat of our car, get out of the car at the surgeon's office and then to get onto the medical table for my exam. I felt like I had run a 5K road race.

When I got to my appointment, my doctor checked my incisions and my drains. The purpose of the drains was to remove excess fluid from the surgical areas, so that my body would not swell up. They also allowed for better healing. My doctor told me I was healing well and I needed to leave my drains in a little bit longer. I complained to him that I felt odd, because everything hurt, especially my right arm and yet so much of my body felt numb. He told me that my right arm was badly bruised and I needed to keep it elevated and allow my body to resorb the collected blood. We left his office satisfied that I was healing as he expected, but realizing that I had a long way to go.

Let me add here a little gem for those of you considering massive surgery. A good friend of mine had warned me before my surgery to buy a raised plastic toilet seat, so I would not have to bend so far when using the commode. That one suggestion made the difference in helping me adjust and was a real life saver. There was no way I could have bent down and gone to the bathroom, in my condition, without one of those seats. It was still quite painful and awkward for me to lift myself up and on to the toilet seat, but at least it was doable.

This brings me to an issue that came up for me on the fifth day after my surgery, that of constipation. This topic is rarely discussed much in books talking about surgery. Constipation is very common and happens to most people when taking pain medications. Believe me when I tell you that it will most likely happen to you, too, and it's much better to consider it ahead of time and plan for it.

I had not been eating a lot at first, but as the days went on and I could eat more regular meals, I began to feel bloated and unable to have a bowel movement. My abdomen was all sutured up and hurting and I was wearing an elastic compression garment that covered my entire chest and mid-section from under my breasts to below my hips. This garment caused my breathing deep, full breaths to be quite difficult and kept me feeling all bound up. After I began eating more food, it became even harder for me to breathe deeply and my mid-section felt very strained.

I had been taking all the bowel softeners the doctor had prescribed and my own supply of H2GO, Active Magnesium tablets. However, those were not enough at first and it looked like I needed extra help. So, one day I became so worried that we called my surgeon. He advised me to increase my dosage of stool softeners, drink prune juice, eat lots of prunes and do whatever I had to in order to go to the bathroom. That led to another shopping excursion for my husband and a new regimen for me. Fortunately, it worked well and relief came quickly.

I want to share with you what my basic routine was early on. During the first couple of weeks after my surgery, I would get up each night needing to use the bathroom, sleep in till 8 or 9am, take my pain meds as directed, move in and out of sleep during the morning, listen to healing and meditation tapes and try to eat something while lying down. I tried to limit how many times I got up, because each time it was such a big ordeal and took a lot of time and energy and really zapped my strength.

Besides being in a lot of pain I found the early recuperation period very challenging, to say the least. For someone like me with a very compulsive personality about being organized and in control of everything around me, I had to learn to just stay put in the recliner and let everything else go. I had to forget about all the dirty dishes piling up in the sink, reviewing the mail, reading a book or the newspapers, or any of my normal daily routines. However, being in so much pain and feeling incapacitated, doing very little was much easier for me to accept and I was able to let it all go.

I went for my next follow up appointment on Friday, nine days after my surgery. My doctor thought my inner, upper arms appeared swollen and he tried to drain them, but couldn't get much fluid out. This issue was directly related to the incident with my health care aid injuring my arm. He told me to start using warm compresses and keep elevating my arm, and gave me an appointment for the following Tuesday. Although this appointment was a little easier than the last one, it still took a lot out of me, and by the time I left his office and got into our car, I hurt all over.

Little by little, some parts of my body began to feel better, but others felt even more uncomfortable. At the next 2 appointments, he removed 5 of my drains, my pain pump, my belly sutures, and left in the resorbable sutures, one drain in the right back and the compression belt. The doctor said that now I could shower.

That weekend, after figuring out how to shower, my husband noticed a sore area on my tailbone that concerned him and 2 triangular areas on my inner crotch that did not look normal. Since I could not bend or move very much, I had to depend on my husband to inspect everything for me. My husband felt they were not healing appropriately, so we called the doctor and we were told he was in surgery for the next 2 days and he could see me on Friday. The nurse advised us to place Bacitracin, an antibacterial ointment, on the areas in question and cover them lightly with sterile gauze and tape.

Let me mention here that up until this entire surgical process, I had been an extremely modest woman. However, out of necessity I had to change my attitude and become much more open and less self-conscious, which was important for my ultimate survival and best interests.

When I saw my doctor on the next Friday, he removed my last drain and looked at the areas of concern and reassured us that they were healing fine. He told us to keep placing Bacitracin or Neomycin on all of them and cover them with gauze for protection. He said that the inner thigh, triangular area was commonly the slowest to heal, and required additional care and attention. He said that the inner thigh, triangular tissue tends to break down, heal, break down, and heal over many times, until they eventually closed up when they were fully healed. He said that if there was ever to be any complication from my kind of surgery, it was there.

I was also told to start moving around, to get up and walk, and to begin to stand up straighter and stretch out my skin, so I was not walking hunched over. He basically wanted me to start using my body more. He reassured me that I would not pull open any incisions and that everything was healing well and could withstand my normal movements.

I must tell you, that I was quite worried and stayed that way for a long time. My crotch areas hurt the most, felt the most stretched, felt very vulnerable to infection and did not look like they was healing correctly. The right side did slowly but surely fill in and heal, in a couple of months, but the left side took a very long time. I was also in moderate discomfort and really had very little energy to do much of anything. Therefore, I didn't move around much and stayed pretty inactive and recliner bound.

On the following Tuesday, I still thought it was healing too slowly and worried constantly about stretching my inner thighs and causing additional damage. When I look back now, I know that at the time, I felt like I was doing exactly what he told me and as much activity as possible. I walked inside and around the outside of our house as much as I could. However, truthfully, I realize that my skin hurt so much and it felt so painful when I stretched a lot, that I was over cautious and did not move my body nearly enough nor did I walk straight enough.

I can definitely say that my current back problem that developed, in relation to my gait, was created during this time. So my advice, for those of you undergoing any cosmetic surgery, is to push yourself to your limits and past your fear and discomfort. It's a matter of "pay now or pay later"! I can assure you that later will be harder on your body, more time consuming and create additional chronic burdens for you.

On my 3rd week post-operative appointment, my surgeon told me with a big smile:" You have the body of a 20 year old and now I can even bounce a quarter off of your stomach". This made my husband laugh, but truthfully, I was in such pain and fear of what was happening with my healing, that his comment did not seem very funny to me at the time. I hoped that I could appreciate his comment when this was all behind me. It was obvious that he was extremely pleased with his surgical results and the state of my healing. He said my upper, inner legs were contoured pretty much as he had planned and shaped nicely, and that the incisions were high enough that I could wear a skirt and barely notice any scarring.

I trusted him and knew that he treated many patients and his judgment was probably realistic and true. I was also pleased that the final results were esthetic to him, but at that moment, lying on his medical table in pain, I was more concerned with why my inner thigh area was healing so slowly and why I was still in so much pain.

I realized then and feel that it is very important to mention here that surgeons DO NOT view the surgical process the way a patient does. Surgeon's simply look at the physical result and "their handiwork", while a patient experiences the result, physically, emotionally, spiritually and everything in between. It would be very nice if it was different, but it just is the way it is.

I began to be more diligent and do everything he suggested. I did my best to go for more walks around my house and my yard each day. I put Bacitracin on the open surgical sites 3 times a day with gauze, I showered regularly, I moved my body as much as I possibly could, and I kept trying to sleep upstairs in our bed.

In time, I noticed that my energy had returned and I did not tire out as quickly. I did get sore and uncomfortable, but for the most part I felt fine. I began to get restless and bored and what surprised me the most was that I would have these unexpected moments of emotional outbursts of anxiety, sadness and fear. I want to call them "Post Traumatic Surgical Stress", but perhaps that is being too dramatic. I am sure anyone undergoing that much surgery and having a long recuperation period, has many emotional moments filled with fear, doubt and insecurity mingled with joy and relief.

It was amazing to me when, in time, my inner thighs started losing some scabbing and there were areas underneath of my own skin knitting together, and at the end stages of healing. The human body is truly remarkable! To have the experience of having so much of my body cut up and sewn back together and then to have my body knit itself together, and be ready to be stretched naturally again is an incredible experience.

One of my most recurring and haunting thoughts during the next four weeks was that I was the one that had CHOSEN to have all of the five surgeries done at the same time. I distinctly remember about one week post-surgery, waking up after having a bad dream and crying out loud one night; "What the hell was I thinking"?!!" I had never considered or could have ever imagined just how dependent and helpless I would be, until I lay there in my living room feeling so vulnerable and like an invalid.

The three and a half weeks that I took off from work to recuperate turned out to not be enough. I had to change my plans and take off three and a half additional weeks in order to be able to heal well enough to get back to work and onto a part time, low stress schedule. Never did I imagine just how difficult it would be for me.

In October, seven weeks after the surgery, I was feeling very impatient with just how long the entire healing process was actually taking. I could move around more and do more puttering around my house, but when I would follow my doctor's advice and stretch my body, I would feel very sore later that day and exhausted the next day. I was completely off all the strong pain meds since 3 weeks post-surgery, but I needed Advil during the day and Tylenol PM in order to sleep at night. I could only sit one way, lay one way and stand one way. There were many parts of my body, especially where the actual incisions were, that still hurt too much to do anything. I had areas that were totally numb and unable to move or function effectively. My most uncomfortable areas were my entire crotch, my inner thighs, and my backside along my upper buttocks. I could not bend or reach the floor, but my arms could finally reach behind my back to shower, wash myself and my hair, and to get myself dressed.

I clearly saw more improvement every day, but when I would increase my physical activity one day, I noticed a slight relapse the following day, where I would feel so sore that I could not do much at all.

What became the hardest thing for me to accept was my intellectually being ready "to move on" and get back to work with my regular activities and work load, but actually being too worn out and tired after what seemed to me to be very little activity. When I complained to a friend, she told me that when she was pregnant, she had undergone an extremely difficult pregnancy that included many months of severe nausea and inability to get around, and becoming bedridden and wishing she could just deliver early, but knew that she could not. It helped to hear of other people's struggles and that in life we have to allow the process to happen and be patient and accept where we are at each moment.

It became so clear to me just how naïve I had been when I made my plans thinking everything would be easy and that I would be able to get right back to my regular life schedule. I am grateful that although I had been unrealistically optimistic in the early planning stages, that when things went awry, I was able to be flexible, stay strong and have an enormous amount of patience and faith.

As a food addict in recovery, one of the more challenging parts for me was that my physical pain and need to be in a reclining position for so long, kept me quite limited in my eating abilities. Immediately after the surgery and for the first week or so following, I was not very hungry and seemed to get by with very small amounts of food and whatever my husband could help feed me while I was almost fully reclined. For many weeks during the early recuperating phase, I had to lay back in the lounger-recliner to allow for healing and to prevent undo pain and suffering for myself. It was extremely uncomfortable for me to even get up slightly in order to eat. I wanted to eat, but physically sitting up was an impossibility.

On October 12th, I wrote: "Today as I lay here still unable to return to work or really even get up and do anything on my own, I have been thinking what a modest person I have always been until now. As of the day of my surgical appointment, I was forced to lose all my modesty, since I had to depend completely on others for my actual survival. My never having been in a hospital for any type of surgery and never being cut by a surgeon's knife, gave me no experience as to what I would undergo or have to deal with post operatively. How naïve and clueless I was! I do not think anyone can truly prepare themselves 100% for a surgery of this kind, unless they have already had some type of invasive surgery, requiring a hospital stay."

In January, when it was four months post-surgery, I began to feel more settled in my body, and get a sense of what my final status would be. My food plan was divided into 5 to 6 small meals and I noticed my weight stabilizing. I still needed a "diet steak day" about once a week, in order to keep me in the lower range of my goal weight. I felt troubled by needing a steak day so often, but felt that after all I had done to achieve my weight loss and the price I had paid to have my desired body, that it was worth it and I owed it to myself.

One of the side effects from my surgery is my having moderate discomfort after eating or drinking too much of anything. My surgeon had tightened up my stomach so much, that as soon as it gets distended, even the slightest amount, and I feel intense pressure. I also have residual feelings of bloating and a reoccurring problem with digestion issues. It seems no matter what I have done to correct this, it remains a constant in my life and my only realistic option is to accept it and deal with it the best I can. When the bloating becomes too much, a steak day can sometimes alleviate the discomfort and take off the added weight.

After a few months, I was able to begin my rebounding again, every morning after I weighed myself, even though my body felt stiff and immoveable. I discovered that the more I stretched myself, the easier it became. Over time, I could even go a little longer and move more freely and with greater flexibility. I imagine it would be like this with any exercise. I even decided to try some Zumba and belly-dancing classes, but it felt too odd and unsettling when I jumped around, since so much of my body was still numb and felt like a dead weight in my mid-section.

Since I have always disliked exercise finding it very demanding and challenging for me, I allowed myself to take it very slowly. I decided that it was important for me to continue my daily stretching and rebounding regimen and prepare myself for when I could take on a more intense workout. I am sure that if you like exercising or want a faster physical recovery that you would want to plan more exercise than I did.

My daily stretching regimen was helping me to accomplish a personal goal of making my basic movements easier and my suture lines more flexible and comfortable. It was also important for my body to reestablish its balance and to work on keeping my posture more erect.

As time went on I found that I could stretch my arms and body better and that my appetite returned full force. I felt so much better and therefore had more food choices. This was the time I had to be extremely diligent and careful, since I could easily get myself into trouble.

Here is a quote from my journal written in May: "It has been about 8 months since my surgery and I am thinking about when I made the big decision to have all four/five major surgeries done together. It's almost embarrassing to acknowledge how utterly clueless I was as to the possible consequences and how long it would take for me to recuperate. Imagining the actual process of having my skin cut, peeled away from my muscles, having the excess skin cut away, and then realigned and sewn up, was just something I was unable to do at the time."

Having had no past experience to draw upon, I did not know what the physical, emotional, or spiritual consequences would be for me. Intellectually I understood the process of surgical preparation, undergoing anesthesia, and the need for a reasonable recuperation period. I had the expectation that since I was a very healthy woman and an excellent healer, I would therefore have less risk, and a very high chance of success. My surgeon had even told me this at my preliminary consultation. However, I have since learned that being a healthy person does not negate the reality that surgery in and of itself has consequences and side effects for everyone."

In retrospect, it seems that was all I could grasp and get my head around at the time. So it does not surprise me that after all the drains were removed and all my sutures were gone and the surgical areas were mending, and I was still having moderate discomfort, feeling disabled and unable to sit correctly in a chair, and only able to sleep on my back, propped up with pillows on all sides and laying in one fixed position, that I wondered if I had made a huge mistake. It was then that I fully understood that I had "taken on more than I had bargained for", and there was no going back.

I had been prepared for a short term, lingering discomfort as a result of surgery, but definitely not for all the rest that I encountered. When I finally realized the possibility that I might have a long term aching in my body, continued discomfort after eating, and physical limitations of movement, I had many moments when I seriously regretted what I had done.

I knew that I could not go back in time and that I had to accept my physical status and learn to do the best with what I had. I chose to marvel at the fact that my surgeon had removed almost 4 pounds of skin from my body and to really appreciate just how much firmer my body looked. I found that in order to stay positive, I had to focus on my newly contoured body shape and remember my original reasons for wanting to have the surgery done in the first place. That attitude kept me from getting stuck in any negativity or anger that I could have easily gotten caught up in.

It was at this time that I noticed that some of my clothes fit much tighter since my surgery and that my weight had gone up between 3-6 pounds from my thinnest HCG weight. This was disheartening, since I had assumed that all my clothes would fit looser and I would have even lost a few pounds after the surgery.

When I went for one of my follow-up appointments, I questioned my doctor about this and he told me that it was from my body's inflammation and swelling and that it would change once I was fully healed, could stand erect, and could really determine how my clothes fit. He reminded me that it would take about 12-18 months for my scarring to fully mature and my body to adjust. When I asked him about the uncomfortable and unsettling numbness that I still had in my body, he assured me that almost all of my numbness should go away within 18 months.

While I waited for my body to heal, I spent a lot of time thinking and wondering and really worrying about what my future would be like. That was when my realization came that we each get so used to our bodies and how they usually "feel", that for the most part, we really take them for granted. We become aware of what makes them hurt or what makes us become "uncomfortable", but not many of us will stop and notice when we feel "comfortable" or what feels "normal" for us. It is only when we are injured or sick, that we are forced to become truly aware of the way our body feels or how it relates to our daily activities.

So, when we are involved with some trauma or have surgical intervention, like, cosmetic surgery, we do our best to plan for all our physical needs and concerns that may come up. This can include medications to help with healing, special tools and home care aids we may need, and post-operative devices that can help our recuperation. However, we can never truly know ahead of time, exactly how our bodies will respond to the actual insult, what specific issues may develop for us or what we will "feel" like. Unless we have already been through a similar experience, we cannot be expected to really predict what it will be like for us.

As for me, I had envisioned my extreme joy to rid myself of the ugly sagging skin and the pain that I experienced from the chafing between my thighs when I walked. I had fantasized what it would be like to not have painful, ugly sores or unsightly stretch marks on my body that were visible to all. I dreamed what it would be like to not need to limit my physical activities or what choices of clothing I was able to wear, and I had prayed that all those limitations would be a thing of the past. I honestly spent very little time imagining what I would feel like being cut up and sewn back together. I would expect that this is what most patients do undergoing this process.

It is now 5 and ½ years post-surgery, when I had expected to be feeling "normal" and able to function as I used to. However, I still feel like I have a tight vice around my body, from my stomach and mid-section all around to my back, ALL THE TIME. It feels worse than having a girdle on, because I can never take it off to let me feel relaxed and comfortable or what used to be "normal" to me.

When I shower or bathe or touch certain areas of my body, I feel absolutely nothing. I occasionally feel soreness in my inner arms when I stretch to reach something, put moderate pressure against the scarring or when I do my daily exercises. Whenever I stretch or pull against my inner thighs, I can feel the scarring pulling and a slight aching. I feel almost no sensation and am still extremely numb around my hips and back.

This causes my sense of my body and how I relate in the world around me to always be in question. I cannot even enjoy a simple loving, human hug or tender touch the way I used to or the way my body was meant to. The surgery has changed the physical sensations I feel related to any sensual or sexual touch, making them almost non-existent, depending on what part of my skin is involved. This was not one of the side effects that I expected or was warned about by my surgeon. Perhaps, I am a very "hypersensitive" person, but I have seriously wondered if any of it could have been predicted ahead of time by more pre-testing.

As I try to understand what has happened to me that resulted in this residual numbness, my thoughts drift back to the "black box" that I opted to have placed during my surgery. I am referring to the Lidocaine anesthetic pump that was released thru a line into my stomach and mid-section, as an adjunct to help minimize any post-operative pain. I wonder if having so much lidocaine going into my surgical wounds for a long period of time created tissue or nerve damage that led to my still being numb years past what my surgeon told me to expect. It seems that this numbness will most likely be with me indefinitely.

When I expressed this concern to my surgeon, he vehemently denied that there was any connection to the "black box" or his surgical technique to my "residual numbness" status.

He explained it all away by calling me an unusually hypersensitive patient.

There may not be a definite answer to this, but it's certainly something for you to inquire about if you decide to have cosmetic surgery.

Another side effect that occasionally disturbs me is some annoying, residual nerve issues in my upper arms that seem to crop up when I least expect it. This issue in addition to being frequently bothered by the noticeable scarring on my upper, inner arms and the toll that this part of the surgery took on me has me regretting that I had my arms cut at all.

When I had my second consultation with my doctor, I shared with you that we had a discussion about my arm surgery and what it would be like. I know that I asked the proper questions, but it was definitely hard for me to imagine what it would be like "post-surgery" not having full extension of my arms at the same time as not being able to move the rest of my body. Somehow in my head, all I could think about was how it made common sense to combine everything and not have to go thru surgery twice or miss extra work. It seems that I added my arm surgery to the plan, thinking it was the rational thing to do, while ignoring some important facts. I find it is amazing how we can talk ourselves into doing something that may not really be in our best interests. How easy it can be to allow our rational mind or our imagination or our emotions to overcome the reality of a situation and our own common sense.

If anyone is considering upper arm surgery, I think it is important to really look at what your arms look like and how much excess skin there actually is. The consequences of the arm surgery will leave you with long, ugly, visible, red scarring on both of your inner arms that may look much worse than the original sagging you had. That was true for me.

However, the most difficult side effect for me has been the tight "tummy tuck" and "butt lift", leaving me always feeling stretched and pulled as if I was wearing a sewed on girdle 24 hours a day. I am constantly in a little discomfort and having to adjust how I do the simplest of things every day. My suggestion for those of you who lost lots of weight and are planning a "tummy tuck" and "butt lift", is to be fully aware that trading the physical problem of excess skin may be replaced by another, possibly more annoying problem. I believe the real key is to know as much as you possibly can ahead of time, prepare yourself well and be honest with yourself as to what you can live with and accept when it is all over.

When I realistically assess my entire process, I most likely would have still chosen 2 or possibly 3 of the surgeries, but I would have at least done them at 2 separate times. It is important for me to keep remembering that much of my personal experience and post-surgical issues stem from my prior metabolism problems and my own physical constraints. I have heard many people tell me of their own post-operative issues after their cosmetic surgeries, including stomach stapling and the lap band, and how varied each of them have been. I have realized that the reality is that every person will end up with their own issues to contend with. We are all individuals and as long as we do our best to be fully prepared, the rest remains to be seen and experienced. You will never know for sure until you do it.

I have since gone back and talked with my surgeon about all my post-surgical issues. He seemed surprised and suggested that I was a highly sensitive woman who experienced things more intensely. Now, when I begin to feel any regret or wish things were different, I make myself stop and compare my pre-surgical photos with my current, firm, beautifully shaped body and decide to feel grateful for how wonderful I look.

My advice to anyone considering major changes to their body is to be fully prepared as to what you are getting yourself into and be sure to choose your surgeries carefully, weighing in all possible outcomes and consequences. Be sure to talk with many others who have already gone thru that exact treatment and what their experience was before, during and most definitely after. Be sure to fully consider all the possibilities, especially the unforeseen and unexpected ones, BEFORE you allow any surgeon to cut on your precious body. Remember, you may not end up with the exact results you had expected or dreamed about.

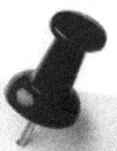

In the past, when my food addiction was at its worst, I used to be a "sleep eater". I would wake up at night, go downstairs to the kitchen, eat for a while in a fog and return upstairs to bed.

CHAPTER 22

Dealing with Insomnia Complicated by Food Addiction

Now is a good time for me to share a little more about my sleeping difficulties. For 3½ to 4 years prior to my surgery, when I started Menopause, I began to have a real problem with insomnia. I would have these bouts of insomnia off and on and I dealt with it by reading in bed, listening to meditation tapes, and trying my best to go back to sleep by cuddling with my pillow. However, after my surgery, I did not have the same ease of movement and ability to just cuddle back in my bed and go to sleep.

I noticed during my post-operative period, where I could only eat very little during the day, that when I would wake up at night, I would feel hungry and want to eat. For me when I do not get enough sleep at night, I become overly weary and can experience what I interpret as food cravings and a need to eat in order to sleep. When this happens, I have an urge to want to wander around my house searching for something to eat. When I first came home from the hospital and felt so bad, I had no problem. However, as my body healed and I could move around more, I found that I had to force myself to stay in bed and wait till the morning.

In the past, when my food addiction was at its worst, I used to be a "sleep eater". I would wake up at night, go downstairs to the kitchen, eat for a while in a fog and return upstairs to bed. In the morning, I would have no clear memory of it, but there were dishes in the sink and food stains on the front of my pajama top. It was a pretty difficult and humiliating time of my life and I never want to go back to that kind of behavior ever again.

Before my surgery, I had a discipline of writing out my food plan for the day. I would eat a small meal in the morning, a little larger meal at lunch, a small, mid afternoon snack and a moderate sized dinner. Then, before I went to bed, I would have a small snack. That food plan worked well for me for a long time.

However, after my surgery, I found that I could not eat very much in the morning and I had to eat very small portions at meal times, because my surgeon had removed all my excess skin and made my sutures so tight that there was very little give in my stomach or chest. Although he told me to stretch out my body every day, the incisions hurt so much and I was afraid that I would tear them or create a split, that I did not do a lot of stretching. As I wrote earlier, I was told that after my incisions healed, my body would be able to stretch more and I'd feel more comfortable.

Well, sleeping during this healing period, when I could only lay on my back, was very troublesome. My body would get quite uncomfortable and sore after a few hours, and I would wake up. My pain medications helped somewhat, but I was still restless and looking for ways to relax and get thru the long nights. Being unable to do much, I would get bored a lot and the more I healed, the more I thought about food.

I discussed this problem with my FA sponsor so we could review my past food plans and figure out what might work best for me. I knew that I could not go back to eating the 3 moderately large meals that my FA friends ate and that I used to eat when I first joined FA, since that was what caused me to regain my weight in the first place. It was just too much bulk for me at each sitting. In addition, as I already mentioned, I had so much tightness in my stomach and mid-section from the surgery that I had to be extremely careful with the types of food and the amount of bulk I ate at each meal.

There were also the changes that had occurred to my metabolism, since I entered Menopause. Not only did I have less physical activity in my life, but my body's daily nutritional needs had changed. I had heard women complain constantly about how much slower their metabolism has become once they got into Menopause, but when it happened to me, it seemed so much more traumatic for the "once fat, now thin woman", that I had become.

I wanted to follow my surgeon's advice to eat "lots of protein", and I wanted to follow my "Weight Loss Cure", Phase 4 plan, but ultimately, I had to decide for myself what I could honestly eat and how much my body could handle. I had my FA sponsor to work with, but it was "new territory" for her and she did the best she could. My trying to juggle different programs was certainly a huge challenge, but I was committed to both the FA and "Weight Loss Cure" programs. I did whatever it took to stay "Abstinent" and treat my body and my health with the utmost of care. I felt that I also had the "Weight Loss Cure's" diet steak day as a fallback position, whenever I found myself gaining weight.

In the first year or so, it seemed in order to stay thin and keep my weight stable; I had to follow one diet steak day a week, because I found myself gaining more than 2 pounds. I had hoped that need would eventually change and I could find a more consistent food plan, that would keep me at an acceptable maintenance weight without having to turn to a diet steak day so often. I am pleased to say that I have been successful and able to do so.

It is now over five and a half years post-surgery and my maintenance weight is slightly higher than my original HCG weight and I still cannot wear some of my pre-surgery clothes. My body shape has remarkably improved, but my waist is a little larger due to all the stretching of skin and body reshaping. Most of my mid body is still partly numb and uncomfortable. As I already mentioned, it actually feels like I am wearing a tight girdle all the time and can be very disturbing and unsettling. Living with the numbness continues to be extremely annoying and difficult in many ways, in addition to being a negative reminder of the lengths I went to for my "dream."

However, I do appreciate my final surgical results and I continue to love seeing my flat stomach on a thin, svelte body. Having to endure some discomfort from the bodies stretching and having a constant numbness does create times of regret and questioning for me, but the bottom line is that my list of pros outweighs my list of cons. I really love having a nice firm body that is very attractive and slim, and I have found an acceptable, stable maintenance weight and food plan that I can live with and enjoy.

CHAPTER 23

Regrets

This chapter is devoted to the honest, nitty, gritty facts that are rarely written about in these types of books.

Although I try to live by the motto "do not regret the past nor wish to shut the door on it" from my 12 Step training; the truth for me is, that there are definitely things I would have done differently had I either had more specific information beforehand, understood fully the consequences of my actions in foresight, or could go back and change some of my prior decisions.

- ¤ I have decided to include this list for all my readers, in order to help you consider them and avoid many of your own regrets later on.
- ¤ I wish I had tried the "Weight Loss Cure" many years ago, before I wasted so much time and energy on everything else.

  In reference to my "Reconstructive", Cosmetic surgery, I wished I had really, fully understood what the post-operative consequences of these surgeries would be like for me and what limitations they would cause. (It has been 5 and 1/2 years since 8/20/08, and I still have some daily discomfort. I am still numb in a large mid-section of my body, I still have abdominal, "stretching pain', when I eat a regular sized meal at one sitting, like most of my FA friends do, and if I drink too much liquid, my belly bulges out and hurts.)

- I would have done much less of the surgery at one time and I would have chosen not to do some of the surgery at all.

- I would have anticipated that my "protecting" the surgical areas and compensating for it when I walked and sat, would lead to my upsetting the delicate balance that my body had been aligned to and was comfortable functioning with.

- Specifically, after the surgery I had to use special pillows to sit, I had to lean when I walked, I did all I could to protect my inner thighs from stretching out too much, and I would sleep fully on my back elevated by many pillows. So basically I completely changed how I was used to functioning in the world. These changes caused my "gait' to be thrown off and led to other spine and back "corrections".

- I believe that, if my surgeon or someone else had warned me about all this and I had been better prepared, I may have been able to prevent some post-operative pain and the resultant limitations that I have experienced since my surgery.

MY HOPE AND INSPIRATION FOR YOU

Before you feel at "wits end and ready to die fat", give yourself a "Gift" and try the "Weight loss Cure"!

This has been a story of how a once fat, now thin recovering food addict was able to get the rest of her unwanted, ugly fat off of her body and keep it off.

I was a food addict working a rigorous 12 Step FA recovery program. I tried many suggested food plans given to me by my sponsors and many other well-meaning FA members, but was still unable to get rid of the resistant, abnormal, fat deposits, also called "Cellulite". I remained overweight and looking and feeling different. My excess, unwanted fat hung firmly around my midriff and thighs and belly, and seemed resistant to any dietary means that had worked for the majority of the other FA members.

Since joining FA, I have been very committed and have tried every suggestion I was given. However, when my weight and remaining fat would not budge; I had to seek more extreme measures.

Gratefully, I was eventually led to "The Weight Loss Cure" where using my disciplined structure of FA, I was able to utilize and follow Dr. Simeone's protocol, that this book was taken from. I was able to lose my excess and unsightly abnormal fat, and to FINALLY find a food plan and protocol for maintaining my weight loss. At last I feel successful and content with my body and my food.

I know that most FA'ers and many food addicts can find weight loss and success with other regimens, but if you feel like you have tried it all and have never been truly successful, do not give up until you try this. Finally getting rid of your ugly cellulite around your hips, thighs, derriere and midriff or wherever it is stuck will make you feel quite beautiful. You will be glad you did not give up.

Summary

Following the weight loss cure program was definitely a serious commitment and I knew that I was most assuredly ready and willing to do it. I want to stress how important I think it is for anyone planning to do this, to follow the Phases exactly as outlined. I truly believe that it will work for anyone if they follow it fully. I also welcome anyone to e-mail me and share your experience as you go through the process. I know you will be completely satisfied and have your thinner body as a result.

Summary Personal Advice

Note to those of you that are "thinkers", "questioners", "intellectualizers", or the "conscientious types". This advice is directed at all of those pedantic people who simply must know it all before you tackle anything new and have to read and research a topic fully and be able to understand it all prior to doing anything. I sympathize with you and understand you completely.

After I read Kevin's book titled, "The Weight Loss Cure" twice, I knew I was going to pursue the "Weight Loss Cure" as a solution, but I still had so many unanswered questions. I had to go online to check it out and had to call the HCG Medical clinic, until I could locate and download Dr. Simeone's original protocol. Then I had to read it cover to cover, three times in order to understand it. This was wonderful for me and made the difference. Get it and read it! Not only did I understand it and appreciate the doctor's viewpoint and knowledge, but it finally explained to me why I had never been able to have total success with any other diet plan. It explained where my body went off balance, and was different from other people I knew, and it gave me even more faith and hope that I could do it. It allowed me to finally believe that if I would follow it, then it would work for me…and IT DID.

One of the most important statements made was on page 32 of Dr. Simeone's Foreword and Transcript. "The problems of obesity are not as life threatening and perhaps not as dramatic as the problems of cancer, but they do often cause "lifelong suffering". I must say that this statement summarizes my story and my feeling about my entire life. I hope I can maintain my newly found thin body for the rest of my life. I hope when you decide to follow this protocol, you can too.

About The Author

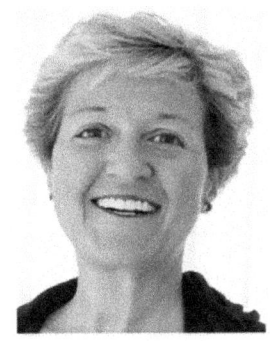

Dr. Susan R. Cushing graduated Cum Laude from Boston College and went on to earn her DMD degree from Tufts University Dental School in Boston, Mass. She had her 1st dental practice in Boise, Idaho where she met and ultimately married her husband Curt and then opened her 2nd dental practice in Pocasset, Mass.

She has long struggled with her weight and her issues around food and has spent many years learning all she could about nutrition, diets, weight control and anything and everything related to it.

In this book, she shares honestly about her past history from childhood to present including her trials and tribulations, challenges and successes. She tells us what finally worked for her and has given her the freedom from the isolation of her fat and food addiction. She tells it like it is and shares her truth very honestly and sincerely.

She lives in Pocasset, Mass. with her loving husband, Curt and her beloved Shih Tzu, Lilly.

You can email your questions and/comments regarding this book directly to Dr. Cushing.

The email address is FatNoMoreBook@gmail.com.

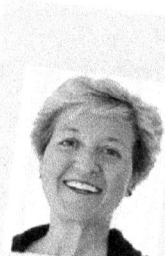
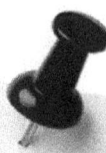

The author of this book is a dentist, not a medical doctor.

Author's Disclaimer

The author of this book is a dentist, not a medical doctor. She is sharing her personal experience, trials and tribulations, successes and failures.

It is strongly advised that before you start any weight loss program, you should consult with a licensed health care provider about your personal medical status for your own safety and optimum success.

Please be advised that doing anything recommended or suggested in this book or related to any specific references she makes in this book must be done at your own risk.

Susan's story is her personal journey. Dates and events are given as accurately as possible. The author has been advised to include this disclaimer due to the litigious nature of our modern world and to suppress any criticism or disappointment from any individual's lack of success or unfilled expectations.

However, with that said, the author strongly believes in the success possible if one follows her suggestions in this book as it honestly affects them and their food and weight problems.

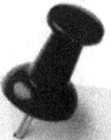

Here is a list of suggestions and suggested products to help you with the HCG process.

Bibliography, Resources and References

- "Pounds and Inches: A New Approach to Obesity", by A.T.W. Simeons
- "The Weight Loss Cure" by Kevin Trudeau
- Also see References in Appendix from Kevin Trudeau's book, The Weight Loss Cure
- The 12 Steps of Alcoholics Anonymous and how it has been interpreted by Food Addicts in Recovery
- "The Secret" by Rhonda Byrne
- "Rethinking Thin" by Gina Kolata
- Here is a list of suggestions and suggested products to help you with the HCG process:
  - Digestive Enzymes (w/meals) - Garden of Life, www.qalabs.com Q-Zyme Ultra
  - www.naturalcures.com
  - Organic Triple Fiber Max- 800-690-9988
  - Alpha Calm (800) 554-6051
  - Whole Food Supplement (www.qnlabs.com)
  - Electromagnetic chaos eliminator- (qline of ependant and biopro for cell phone)

- www.bioprotechnology.com
- www.ewater.com
- www.clarus.com
- Extra Virgin Raw Coconut Oil
- Shower filter (www.ewater.com or www.wellnessfilter.com)
- Candida Cleanse Three Lak- www.123candida.com or www.lifeforeplan.com
- Probiotics- www.qnlabs.com

All products used should have No propylene glycol or mineral oil or sodium laurel sulfate.

- Buy Organic Hair Gel and Shampoo
- Take Vitamin E Daily
- Take Omega 3 Daily
- Use Stevia for a Natural Sweetener
- Take Probiotics
- Buy Organic Beef, Chicken, Veal, Fruits and Vegetables
- H2GO - Lane Laboratories
  [Items can be purchased directly or from www.compassionet.com]

Also, eat dinner by 6 PM. Eating between 5:30 to 6 PM is best. Eat at least 3 ½ hours before bed time.

Overview of Susan's Lifelong Weight Challenge

I have spent a majority of my life trying to get thin. I looked everywhere I could for a way to stop the nagging food cravings and obsession that haunted me and kept me feeling like a prisoner in my life.

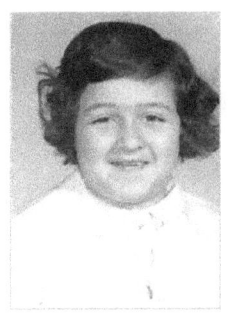
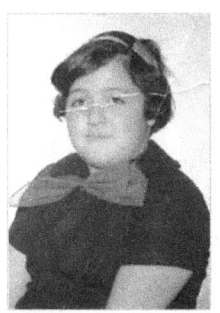
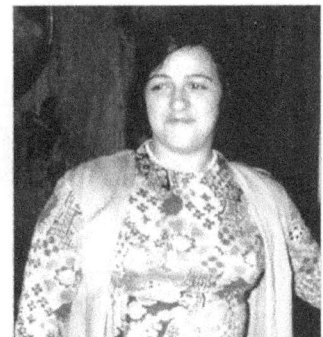
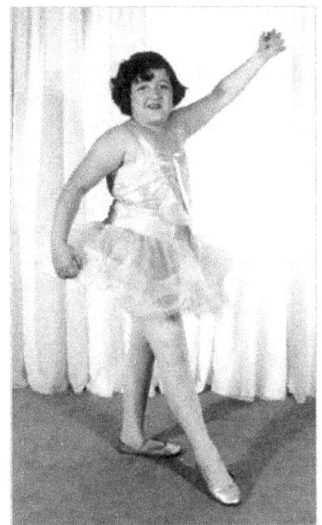
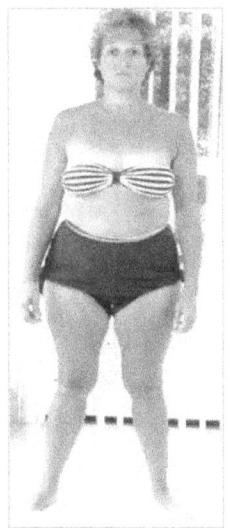

SUSAN AS A CHILD, YOUNG ADULT AND BEFORE HER WEIGHT LOSS SUCCESS

I was a pudgy child, a fat teenager, an obese young adult and a full-figured career woman.

Now, I am a slim, healthy mature woman in recovery from food addiction with extensive personal research to share on what has worked and what has not.

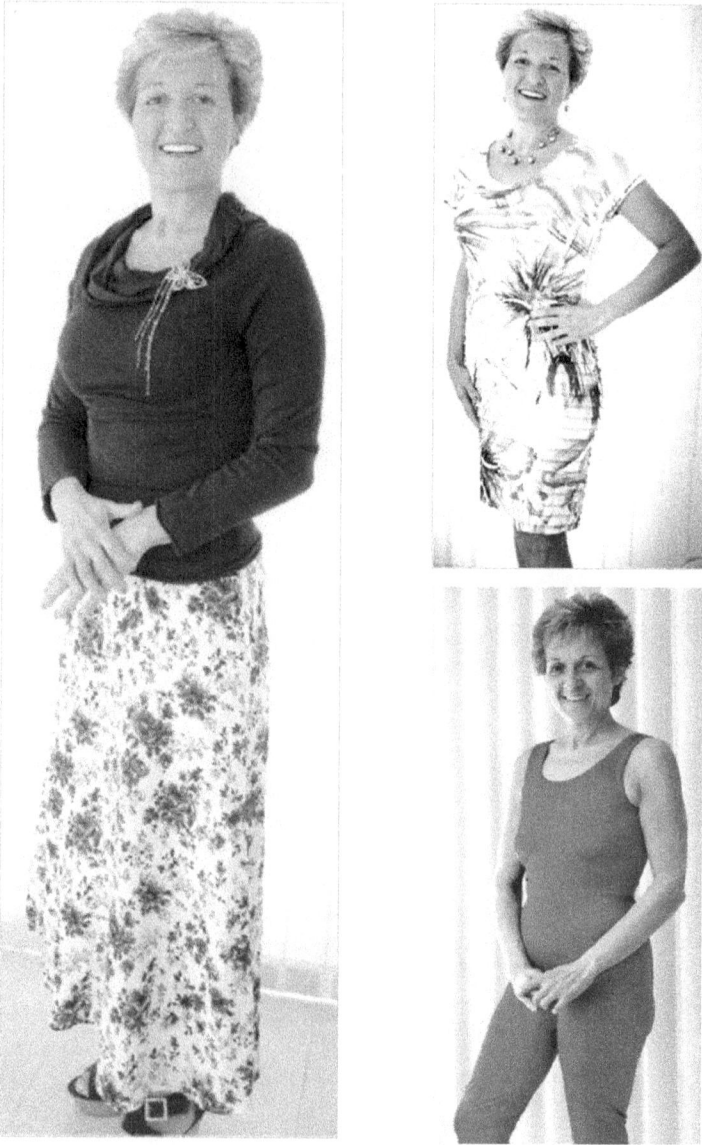

SUSAN AFTER SHEDDING 85 POUNDS AND KEEPING THE WEIGHT OFF FOR OVER SIX YEARS

It has been my lifelong desire to help others and make a real difference in people's lives.

I became a dentist, focusing on cosmetic dentistry and in treating the fearful and phobic dental patient, as one means to this end. As wonderful as this career has been for me and as many lives that I know I have empowered and changed, I do not believe it can hold a candle to my personal journey with food. After all the struggles I have gone through with my weight and food issues, I believe I can improve and empower others' lives by honestly sharing my research and my personal story.

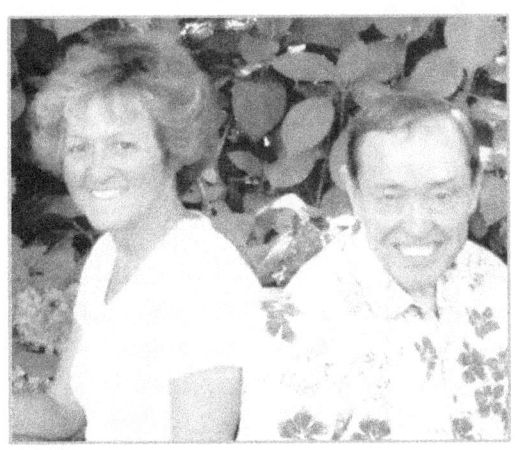

SUSAN WITH HER COMPANION AND LOVING HUSBAND OF 29 YEARS, CURT

This book is not only personal to me. It is also for the thousands of men and women who have been waiting for such a book. This book will help them gain insight and answers they have been wanting and unable to find.

I believe that by honestly sharing all the struggles and successes that I have gone through with my weight and food issues, I will empower others and ultimately improve their lives. I am committed to helping my overweight and possibly addicted fellows out there find their inner peace and slimmer selves.

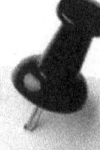

You can email your questions and/comments regarding this book directly to Dr. Cushing.

The email address is FatNoMoreBook@gmail.com

www.ingramcontent.com/pod-product-compliance
Lightning Source LLC
Chambersburg PA
CBHW032112090426
42743CB00007B/324